EX

Prevention & Treatment
Your Personal Guide
to Sports-Medicine

Distributed by
Stackpole Books
Cameron & Kelker Streets
Harrisburg, PA 17105

EXERCISE INJURIES
Prevention & Treatment
Robert C. Cantu, M.D.,
F.A.C.S., F.A.C.S.M.

Stone Wall Press, Inc.
1241 30th Street, N.W.
Washington, D.C. 20007

Published September 1983

Library of Congress Card Number 83-50359
ISBN 0–913276–56–6

7072958

To Rob, Biz, and Jane

Contents

ACKNOWLEDGMENTS

I would like to express my sincere appreciation to Victor Wright Quale, a talented artist, for his superb illustrations, Chris Stackhouse for his fine photographs and Stephanie Chase for posing for many of the these photos. I also wish to acknowledge my appreciation to Human Sciences Press and Norma Fox, Executive Vice-president, and the Callamore Press and Editor Sarah Boardman, for allowing me to use material from *Toward Fitness* and *Sports Medicine In Primary Care* respectfully. Finally, I want to thank my secretary par excellence Pat Blackey, whose skills facilitated the preparation of this manuscript while simultaneously managing a busy neurosurgical office.

Section I
Keys to a Healthy, Active Life

Chapter 1

Conditioning of the Cardiovascular System: A Machiavellian Approach to Health

Niccolo Machiavelli, in *The Prince,* his renowned book about how to achieve and hold power, wrote: "Fortune is the arbiter of half the things we do, leaving the other half or so to be controlled by ourselves."

Machiavelli was concerned with the health of the state, but his wisdom also applies to a healthy body. Fortune dictates to a certain extent our basic health at birth. During the first years of our lives, our health may be partially determined by the care given our body by others—usually parents. Parents dictate what we eat and by their examples—good and bad—affect our personal health habits. Teachers also influence us, as do our classmates, and, sometimes unfortunately, TV commercials promoting various products. But eventually each individual grows older and wiser and exerts increasingly greater control over his or her body. It is at this point that Machiavellian principles of good health can be applied.

Niccolo Machiavelli lived in Florence at the start of the 16th century and served as part of a court where the principal sport seemed to be intrigue, not jogging. But were he to be born again in the 20th century, he would recognize that a prince today would need to maintain good physical fitness to guarantee his survival power. Machiavelli would probably advise his prince to look after his biological clock.

What is a biological clock? It is a time machine, ticking within each individual. This time machine, set before birth, dictates the maximum length of every person's life. One of the most important factors governing our basic health is heredity. We are what our parents make us. We remain alive only while our vital organs function. Although medical science recently has made significant progress in transplanting hearts, kidneys, and other parts of the body necessary to life, we can only survive as long as the least of these vital parts survive.

The sad fact is that people weaken their organs through their individual abuses such as excessive alcohol consumption, cigarette smoking, and the like. In addition, because of lack of physical activity (hypokinesia), people also fail to maintain their body parts in optimum condition to guarantee them not merely long life but also good health. This might be compared to spending $26,000 for a new Porsche and then forgetting to put oil in the crankcase or change the spark plugs every 6000 miles. The Porsche won't run up to its potential on the highway, and you may even blow the engine apart. It will do you no good to know that your dashboard clock is still ticking if one of the pistons has exploded through the oil pan, immobilizing the car. To carry this analogy to its ultimate conclusion, you may be able to afford a new Porsche, but you only get issued one body.

We are never too old to begin a program of cardiovascular improvement. At birth our vascular system is largely free of fatty deposits; but with each day of life, deposits accumulate in our arteries, threatening our health and survival. The English researcher Osborne showed that early signs of disease can be detected in the coronary arteries of children as young as 5 years. Between the ages of 16 and 20, over half the population has atherosclerosis of the coronary arteries. Autopsy studies of Korean War casualties showed that many of our soldiers had very significant arteriosclerosis before the age of 25. No prince would want his army to exhibit such signs of decay, since it would limit their ability to fight and protect him. Machiavelli would probably demand more physical fitness programs for his prince's armies and, further, insist that a better physical education program be established to guarantee their health *before* being called to service.

The research showing early occurrence of coronary artery disease demonstrates the desirability of a total fitness program from cradle to grave. While playing, most young children run because of their natural inclination. As children grow older, they should never stop running—although most do. However, even for those who have abandoned exercise, it is never too late to begin such a program. Heart patients now complete full distance (26-mile, 385-yard) marathons. Recent studies have shown a reduction in previous arteriosclerosis with endurance cardiovascular training. The buildup of plaques deposited in coronary arteries apparently can be reversed. Health and physical fitness can be regained even by those who seem hopelessly out of shape.

What is physical fitness? What are the best cardiovascular exercises? The answers to these two questions are basic to a fitness program. To understand fitness, it is necessary to know a bit about the physiology of exercise, particularly as it involves the cardiovascular system. Let us consider this system, which might be described as the tree trunk of life.

The cardiovascular system, consisting of the heart, arteries, capillaries, and veins, conducts blood containing life-essential oxygen and nutrients to our body cells. The road to vigorous health begins with a fit cardiovascular system. Physically disadvantaged individuals usually suffer from some impairment of their cardiovascular system. Frequently the disruption is sudden and severe, perhaps a major blockage of a coronary artery or a cerebral artery occlusion or rupture. Others may recognize the deterioration of their cardiovascular system by certain tell-tale signs: excessive fatigue, shortness of breath, or chest pain following physical activity. Heart attacks not only kill and disable more people in the Western world than any other affliction, but as affluent life spreads to the non–Western world, the incidence of heart attack climbs there also.

The root cause of cardiovascular impairment is related to family history. A tendency toward heart attack is built into our genes. If our father or mother suffered early cardiovascular impairment, the odds are that we will, too—particularly if we mimic their health habits.

Because we did not select our parents, our biological clock lies outside our initial control. In Machiavellian terms, fortune has arbited its movement. However, knowing about our family's health history will suggest how we might grasp control and dictate our own destiny. Physically disadvantaged people with a family history of cardiovascular disease should begin an exercise program immediately in order to resist the genetic weaknesses they have inherited. This holds true regardless of their age.

One of the great tributes to good health is the Boston Marathon, run each April from Hopkinton to downtown Boston. Thousands of healthy runners participate in this 26-mile event, which usually is witnessed by more than a million people lining the route. Ironically, the Boston Marathon passes through Framingham, Massachusetts, a town of about 70,000 that has been the site of several classic studies of the health of large groups of people.

One recent Framingham study, begun in 1968 and sponsored by the United States Public Health Service, closely followed more than 5,000 residents (2336 males and 2873 females) and focused on heart disease. The study determined that (1) men with (2) elevated cholesterol levels, who (3) had hypertension or diabetes, and who (4) smoked had 10 times more coronary artery disease than average individuals. With these four factors absent, the likelihood of death from heart disease was reduced to one-third the standard risk. Thus, very clearly, the elevation of blood cholesterol, hypertension, diabetes, and being male greatly increased one's chances of heart attack. (After menopause, women are at equal risk for heart attack as males the same age.)

We should pause briefly to discuss cigarette smoking because it is so important to our health—or lack of health. Cigarette smoking has been identified as a principal cause of certain types of cancer, but smokers stand an even greater risk of suffering a heart attack because of their smoking habits. That smoking significantly increases the risk of heart disease has been proven by epidemiologic studies in the United States, Canada, Great Britain, and elsewhere. In fact, the incidence of sudden death during a heart attack, if it occurs, is nearly 400% greater in cigarette smokers.

There are other factors that increase the risk of heart attack. One such factor is obesity. However, obesity usually is a risk factor only in association with one or more of the other risk factors such as diabetes, hypertension, high blood cholesterol, or inactivity. Usually there is no single reason why people fail to live to the potential programmed on their biological clock, but rather a constellation of reasons.

One other factor is the existence within individuals of emotional stress and the so-called "Type A" personality. A "Type A" individual is characterized as a person who is competitive, excessively ambitious, impatient with delay, compulsive, and never satisfied with any achievement. The findings are far from conclusive, however, as multiple studies in the United States and abroad indicate no correlation between responsibility at work and coronary disease. So perhaps the "Type A" personality is merely associated with other risk factors, such as smoking.

Last among the risk factors most closely identified with heart attacks is inactivity. Professor Jeremy Morris of the British Research Council first drew attention to this fact in 1953 with his report entitled "Coronary Heart Disease and Physical Activity at Work." He studied the incidence of heart disease in London Transport Department workers and found that bus conductors, who averaged 24 trips per hour up and down the winding staircase of the moving double-decker bus, had one-third less heart disease than the more sedentary bus drivers. In 1973 Morris further reported the beneficial effects of leisure-time exercise in 17,000 British civil servants. He concluded: "Habitual vigorous exercise during leisure time reduces the incidence of coronary heart disease in middle-age among sedentary male workers. Vigorous activities which are normal for such men are sufficient. Training of the heart and cardiovascular system is one of the mechanisms of protection against common risk factors and the disease."

More recently, in 1977, Dr. Ralph S. Paffenbarger, Jr., reported that the risk of heart attack is significantly reduced in men engaged in strenuous sports, while "casual" sports seemed to have no beneficial effect. His research involved 17,000 male alumni of Harvard University, aged 35 to 74, who had been studied for 6 to 10 years. Heart attack rates declined among these men in proportion to their degree of physical activity. This trend held true for all ages and for both nonfatal and fatal attacks. The message came through loud and clear: The more calories the men spent in total activity in a week, the less their risk of heart attack.

The magic number at Harvard was 2000. It appeared that 2000 calories expended per week in exercise protected an individual against heart attack.

This protective effect for active men seemed to hold, regardless of whether they had other risk factors, such as cigarette smoking, hypertension, obesity, or a parental heart attack history. Among the strenuous sports affording the most protection were running, swimming, basketball, handball, and squash. "Casual" sports that afforded no protection included golf, bowling, baseball, softball, and volleyball.

Regarding the benefits of daily physical activity, we should reflect on the three regions of the world most renowned for longevity: the Ecuadorian Andes, the Karamoran mountains in Kashmir, and the Agkazia region of the southern Soviet Union. In these regions, people often live to the age of 100 or more, and heart attacks are quite rare. Researchers have noted that diets vary, and partaking of "local spirits" is common amongst the aged. In all three regions, the people assumed they would live to an old age and literally work until they drop. The nature of their work involves heavy physical labor and frequent sustained walking over hilly terrain. These people expend 400 to 800 calories daily while working, and objective physical examination of them shows a very high degree of cardiovascular fitness. Therefore, substantial evidence now exists that cardiovascular fitness, attained either by work or, of necessity, by a formal exercise program for the majority of the modern Western world's sedentary workers, prevents heart attack and increases longevity.

Consider for a moment how the body's cardiovascular system, its tree trunk of life, operates. On earth, our atmosphere contains 21% oxygen. Our body requires a constant supply of this oxygen to survive. Within a few minutes of deprivation, the cells of our body begin to die, starting with our most sensitive organ, the brain.

Our lungs extract oxygen from the atmosphere. Our breathing is controlled automatically by a feedback system from our brain. Specific cells in the brain respond to the blood levels of oxygen, and when the content falls below a critical level, the brain sends impulses through its nerves to the chest wall, diaphragm, and heart. This causes one to breathe more deeply and rapidly, and it is why we seem to get "out of breath" when we run or exercise vigorously. The increased heart rate results in a greater volume of blood being delivered to the lungs to acquire the increased oxygen being supplied.

Our lungs consist of ever-smaller air passages, the major bronchi and smaller bronchioles, and terminate in tiny air sacs known as alveoli. The walls of the alveoli contain fine hairlike capillary blood vessels that are part of the lung's circulation. In accordance with the laws of physics, gasses pass through a permeable membrane, the capillary blood vessel's walls, from a region of high concentration to a region of lower concentration. Thus, oxygen passes from the alveoli to the capillary blood vessels; CO_2 does just the opposite, passing from capillary blood vessels to alveoli.

In the capillary blood vessel, most of the oxygen combines with the protein hemoglobin in our red blood cells. In this form, it is carried away from the lungs to the left side of the heart. From there it is pumped through the arterial system. The arteries branch into smaller and smaller vessels until they end in capillaries, this time in muscles and the other tissues of the body. In this way, oxygen-rich blood is delivered to active oxygen-poor muscles. There the oxygen separates from the hemoglobin under the influence of various environmental conditions, including heat of muscle contraction, acidity, and presence of myoglobin. The net result is that the muscle receives oxygen. The deoxygenated blood returns through the veins to the right side of the heart from which, again, it is pumped to the lungs to repeat the entire cycle (see Figure 1-1).

Muscles exert their work by contracting, or shortening in length. Energy is required to initiate and continue this work, and the source of energy is the food we eat. The major source of short-term energy involves the oxidation of glucose to carbon dioxide and water.

In order to oxidate glucose, the body requires a plentiful supply of oxygen. Without sufficient oxygen, the process halts part way and a toxic substance, lactic acid, accumulates in the muscles and the bloodstream. High lactic acid levels are associated with the sensation of fatigue and eventually lead to the cessation of muscle function. Exercise in which the effort outstrips the body's ability to supply oxygen include underwater swimming and sprinting. These are oxygen deficient, or *an*aerobic, activities as opposed to aerobic activities, where ample oxygen is present. They can be done for only a few minutes before the buildup of lactic acid halts muscle function.

Some people have a greater ability to sustain higher levels of anaerobic work than others. World champions, whether sprinters or distance performers, are *born* as well as made. Training will improve both speed and the ability to incur large oxygen debts, but the potential world record holder possesses a greater potential for anaerobic metabolism before beginning to train. Fortune has arbited this half of his or her athletic ability, to return to Machiavelli's premise.

The other half of the Machiavellian design for health relates to aerobic fitness. The more oxygen one can use per minute, the greater one's ability to perform aerobic-type, or endurance-type, work. Maximal oxygen consumption is the maximum of oxygen one can use per minute. *Fitness is defined in terms of our maximal oxygen consumption, sometimes referred to by physiologists as VO_2 max.* Included in the oxygen transport system that determines this are our lungs, adequate hemoglobin in the blood, an efficient chemical system in our muscles, and the movement of blood by our pump, the heart. Assuming one does not have lung disease and is not anemic, from a practical point of view we can say that one's maximal oxygen consumption is primarily a measure of one's maximal cardiac output. Thus, physical fitness is determined by the efficiency of the heart and is measured by our ability to consume oxygen. This is the answer to the question, what is physical fitness?

Figure 1–1

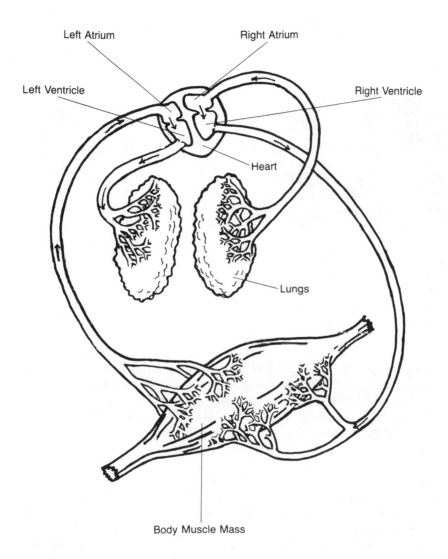

Left Atrium

Right Atrium

Left Ventricle

Right Ventricle

Heart

Lungs

Body Muscle Mass

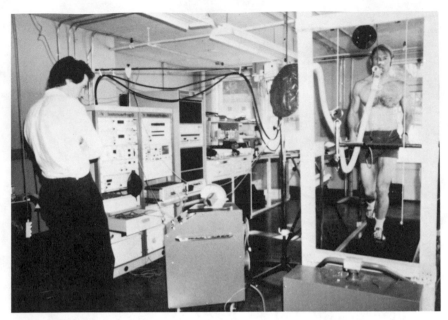

Figure 1–2. Dr. Cantu's maximum oxygen consumption is being tested while he runs on a treadmill.

Thus, maximum oxygen consumption is the measurement of one's greatest capacity to consume oxygen. For any of you who have been in or read about endurance athletics, you must realize that this, the VO_2 max, is a number the athletes seem to focus on. Crew teams and cross-country ski team members, when asked what kind of shape they are in, will answer they are a 74 or 76. In Scandinavia, that number is known as the condition number, and if someone asked you what kind of shape you were in and you replied 80, they would know you were in terrific shape. The highest score ever recorded was 94 by Sveno-Oke Lundbeck, the great Swedish cross-country ski racer. American national cross-country ski team members are in the low 80s. Marathon runner Bill Rogers is 78, and Frank Shorter is 70. Alpine ski racers in the 50s, and the population at large is in the 40s.

To determine maximum oxygen consumption, the best overall assessment of cardiovascular fitness, we must find how effectively muscle is able to extract oxygen from the blood going by. The sum total of the heart, lungs, blood vessels, and muscle interaction is reflected in the maximum oxygen consumption. In Figure 1-2, I am being tested on a treadmill. My nose is blocked, so I am able to inhale through a top valve and exhale through a bottom valve. The exhaled air is continuously monitored for oxygen and carbon dioxide concentration. Knowing the oxygen concentration being inspired, a computer gives a continuous readout of the oxygen consumed. The heart rate is also monitored and fed through an analog digital converter. The computer has eliminated the need for having laboratory technicians to collect exhaled air bags and sample the concentrations of gases in them. Today, most hospitals have the equipment to compute your VO_2 max. We need to consider the next important question: What are the best cardiovascular exercises? The best exercise probably is the one you most enjoy and therefore will be most likely to pursue continuously. But some exercises have certain characteristics that make them more advantageous than others.

First, from a cardiovascular standpoint, the primary objective for good health is sustained vigorous exercise pursued for a length of time sufficient to burn more than 400 calories. The activity should increase the heart rate to approximately 75 to 80% of its maximum potential in order to experience cardiovascular improvement. For most of us, this translates into a pulse rate of around 120–150 per minute to achieve this increased endurance fitness. This also translates, practically speaking, into a 75 to 80% maximal oxygen consumption. To exceed 80% of maximal cardiac output as measured by pulse rate may lead to inadequate oxygenation, that is, anaerobic metabolism and tissue damage. Unless you are a competitive athlete training for victory rather than fitness, this should be avoided.

In reality, most beneficial fitness exercises occur at lower pulse rates. Ideally, exercise will be continuous for 30 or more minutes. You can see why sports such as tennis, with delays between points, or football, with a huddle before every play, rank low as fitness exercises.

The second desirable characteristic for a fitness exercise is that it be rhythmical, with the muscles alternately contracting and relaxing. This implies steady, free flowing movements that, once underway, contain no stops or starts. Such exercises include walking, jogging, running, hiking, cross-country skiing, swimming, bicycle riding, and rowing a boat. In comparison, golf, baseball, football, tennis, and other sports with stop-and-go activity rate poorly.

The third feature of efficient exercise involves the ability to increase the work load as your level of fitness increases. With increased fitness, the same activity that initially caused a pulse rate of 140 may now produce an increase to only 100. Thus, the activity must progressively be made more difficult. This can be accomplished in several ways. You can slowly increase the effort at which you exercise. If you have been jogging a mile in 10 minutes, you can increase your speed to cover that mile in 9 minutes, or 8 minutes. Or you can run further at the same pace. Most beginning joggers, whether consciously or not, employ both methods. Similar changes occur as your physical condition improves in other endurance sports such as cycling or swimming.

Indeed, the final trait of effective exercise is endurance. Exercise should be sustained for at least half an hour and if possible up to 1 hour to produce maximum results. It also should be done at least four days a week and preferably more. The added advantage of exercising every day is only another percent or two of fitness, but your enjoyment may be increased by regular exercise.

The first sign of increased cardiovascular fitness is slowing of the heart rate. This is called *bradycardia* and is experienced both at rest and while exercising. Thus, with a specific amount of exertion, a fit person's heart rate will increase, but it may still be slower than that of a nonfit individual at rest. The second effect of cardiovascular fitness is that the heart pumps more blood with each contraction. The volume of blood pumped per heart beat (medically called *stroke volume*) is thus increased. The heart therefore works more powerfully and efficiently. It can be thought of as loafing along at a slower pace doing the same amount of work, because each contraction is more forceful.

Regular endurance exercise also results in lowering of blood pressure both at rest and with exercise. This means the heart is less susceptible to the noxious influence of the sudden shocks, stresses, and anxiety-provoking situations that confront us daily. In other words, it may be possible to overcome the supposedly bad effect of having a Type A personality if one is fit.

As mentioned before, increased cardiovascular fitness is associated with a decrease in blood pressure both at rest and with exertion. High blood pressure increases the amount of fatty material deposited on the walls of arteries; it literally blows plaque material into the walls of the blood vessels. Increased blood pressure increases the likelihood of a stroke or heart attack. But conversely, increased fitness serves as a deterrent to those conditions.

Frequently a heart attack can be traced to a specific unaccustomed heavy physical exertion or a great anxiety-provoking situation. Each of these situations increases heart rate and blood pressure. If preexisting disease is present, the workload on the heart may outstrip its ability to adequately supply itself with oxygen through its own circulation during *diastole*, the stage in the cardiac cycle when the heart's cavities fill with blood. The result is a heart attack.

Isometric muscle contractions, such as straining to lift a heavy object, can prove especially hazardous to the individual who is not fit, since the rise in blood pressure is disproportionately high. Fit individuals, however, can carry out heavy physical tasks or be exposed to anxiety-provoking situations with very little increase in heart rate or blood pressure. Numerous studies show that people who regularly engage in heavy physical exercise have less increase in blood pressure with advancing years. Too little physical activity, on the other hand, can cause several forms of hypertension.

In several books on the subject of aerobics, Kenneth A. Cooper, M.D., presents a readily understood method of quantifying exercise. He provides charts that give point values for different types of exercises. For example, swimming 250 yards in 5 minutes is worth 2 points, while playing handball for 30 minutes earns 4½ points. Dr. Cooper contends that if people accumulate 30–34 points per week, they can consider themselves physically fit. Dr. Cooper's ideas as to how total physical fitness is achieved are summarized in two basic principles. First, if one exercises 12–20 minutes per day, it must be vigorous enough to sustain a heart beat of 150 per minute. Second, if the exercise fails to reach that level, it must be sustained for a longer period of time to be equally beneficial.

Dr. Cooper also agrees that cardiovascular fitness is realized only by a sustained steady increase in heart rate for periods of at least 30 minutes four times a week. Ideally, the activity should be rhythmic and the intensity increased as fitness improves.

If the objective of exercise is to achieve a sustained increase in heart rate, any activity done at an accelerated rate can be used, from running to vacuuming the floor. However, not all sports meet this criterion. Doubles tennis, for example, rates quite poorly as physical exercise because of the frequent standing around between points. Likewise golf, walking, baseball, football, weightlifting, and even calisthenics do not achieve a sustained increase in heart rate unless maintained for regular periods with short rest intervals. Other sports activities such as downhill skiing, squash, handball, and racquetball generate a moderate level of cardiovascular exercise, but the activity is not continuous. The activities that achieve maximal cardio-vascular exercise levels include running, stationary running, cross-country skiing, roller skiing, swimming, rowing, and cycling.

In summary, the amount of exercise required for good cardiovascular fitness varies with the exercise pursued and how *vigorously* it is pursued. It can be achieved by strenuous continuous exercise periods of as little as 30 minutes' duration three or four times weekly. The same degree of cardio-vascular fitness requires 60 minutes or more three or four times a week if the pursuit is less taxing and is intermittent in nature. Regardless of the activity, one should push it only to the point of breathing deeply, not to being out of breath.

The beneficial effects of endurance training on the normal middle-aged heart include a slowing of the heart rate (bradycardia), increased blood flow to the heart muscle, more efficient and powerful work of the heart muscle, lowered blood pressure, and a decrease in blood fats and their deposit in the body's blood vessels. Machiavelli would appreciate the increased odds this would offer for his prince's survival.

Chapter 2

Life-Style Modification

Now that you are aware that you are responsible for much of your health, let's build on that theme before we embark on specific exercise programs. Today, we in sports medicine are involved not only with the prevention and treatment of injuries, but equally with the promotion of health and fitness through aerobic exercise, appropriate life-styles, and adequate nutrition. We believe the greatest present potential for improving one's health is to be realized in what one does and does not do to oneself. Individual decisions about diet, exercise, and smoking are critical. A recent study at Massachusetts General Hospital disclosed that three out of five hospitalizations could have been avoided if people had taken better care of themselves. While exercise alone is no panacea, the medical evidence is overwhelming that people who live sensibly and keep fit are healthier, feel better, are more productive, have lower absenteeism and better morale at work, and live longer.

Today, we realize that a new direction concentrating on positive health rather than curative treatment must be undertaken. Health cannot be given or brought to the American people; rather, they must learn to take better care of themselves in order to avoid illness and to function at full capacity. Health depends less on medicine than on genetics, life-style, environment, and cultural factors. We must aid people in learning how to help themselves not to require medical attention. Our government realizes that the most potent tool to limit health care expenditures is to concentrate on keeping people healthy rather than on returning them to health after they have become ill. Table 2-1 lists some of the common disease states that are directly attributable to, or whose severity and occurrence are accelerated by, an inadequate life-style.

I liken all of this to a swamp into which the average person may be slowly sinking. A number of years ago, when I still understood what was happening under the hood of my car and worked on it, I walked into a large

Table 2-1
Diseases Attributable to Poor Life-Style

1. Alcoholism and other drug dependency conditions
2. Anxiety states
3. Atherosclerosis
4. Chronic depression
5. Chronic fatigue and lethargy (accompanied by the "let somebody else do it" syndrome)
6. Chronic obstructive pulmonary disease (cigarette smoking)
7. Coronary artery disease
8. Diabetes (adult onset)
9. Emphysema (cigarette smoking)
10. Hypercholesterolemia (excess cholesterol in the blood)
11. Hypertension
12. Marital, family, sexual maladjustments
13. Obesity
14. Osteoporosis (abnormally porous bones)
15. Postretirement involution (decreased mental, physical, and social activity)
16. Stress-related symptoms (including tension headaches, neckaches, back and chest pain, functional abdominal distress)

junkyard, looking for a part for my car. In one corner of this junkyard, I came across an old Rolls Royce, a Silver Cloud that could have been worth $80,000. It was all rusted out and had birds' nests inside of it; the handsewn leather interior was gone and the exterior in utter ruin as well. When you see one of the most magnificent machines that mankind has made in this condition, it is really a rather horrifying experience. You have to ask yourself, how could somebody possibly let a machine as nice as this, which had years of elegant life left, go completely to pieces? But if you think of the Rolls Royce as a nice machine, you cannot begin to compare it to this one that we have all inherited. Owning and operating your body for a number of years, and maintaining it properly, is something I think we should prize highly.

How do we alert ourselves to possible problems? It begins with a personal inventory, a life-style analysis. We should consider our age, sex, occupation, smoking history, diet pattern and quality, current or past regular exercise habits and types, known medical or surgical conditions, current or past regular medications (including over-the-counter drugs), known allergies, and significant family history of illnesses. An occupational history including job satisfaction is also relevant.

Our social history is of utmost importance. This includes the type, location, and number of residences; marital and sexual satisfaction; concerns about children; family planning; hobbies; other interests and activities outside of the job; how much sleep; diet quality and pattern in some detail; type and regularity of exercise; smoking history; alcohol pattern and amount; and drug use or abuse. A part of your life-style analysis should ideally include a thorough physical examination by your physician and basic laboratory blood work. If you are over 35 and have not been exercising regularly or have a family history of heart disease, a stress electro-cardiogram is also suggested.

Life-Style Modification

Now that you have gone through the history, examination, and testing and decided what the risk factors are, laying the groundwork for life-style change necessitates first making sure you understand that the changes must be permanent. A short-term approach with short-term goals just will not be successful. If you are looking for magic, there is none to be found.

There are many positive rewards experienced when a poor life-style is improved. They include improved energy and sense of well-being, a better ability to cope with stress, and automatic eventual control of excess body fat. This is especially true when proper nutrition and aerobic exercise are stressed.

While we are thinking of body fat, I believe it is important to de-emphasize body weight and not concentrate on it. After all, the scale is measuring not just fat but also muscle, bone, and fluid. It is a common and tragic mistake to think that the minute the scale says you have gained weight, you have gained fat. Actually, a thin person doing everything right—following a good aerobic exercise program and eating with proper quality and pattern—may gain weight but still will have lost excess body fat. The muscle mass increase accounts for the added weight. This point must be stressed over and over again, because most are conditioned to think only in terms of weight loss.

Other benefits are a protection against heart attack and the development of adult-onset diabetes. The control of hypertension is improved as is the quality of sleep. Job performance is enhanced as well as one's self-image.

Aerobic exercise by itself appears to be useful in helping to reduce addictive behavior. Many people who have not been able to cut down on alcohol or quit smoking or who have trouble with compulsive eating find the ability after starting an aerobic exercise program. Significant improvement in depression and anxiety states is also seen. Today, many psychiatrists are using aerobic exercise as the primary therapeutic tool to treat depression.

It is exceedingly rewarding to see individuals who used to go home from work and crash in front of the TV now energized and involved in various community tasks and activities. Proper life-style benefits one not only at the personal and family level, but also at the community level.

Finally, an additional reward is a significant reduction in the long-term cost of medical care, since unnecessary illness is prevented or deferred. In

17

Table 2-2
Major Life-Style Risk Factors

1. Abnormal hematologic, metabolic, or other blood or urine tests
2. Cardiopulmonary symptoms or signs
3. Diabetes
4. Family history of cardiac disease and/or hyperlipidemia
5. Family and/or personal history of heavy smoking or alcohol abuse or both
6. "Type A" personality (destructive vs. constructive stress)
7. Hypertension
8. Lack of motivation and ability to improve life-style
9. Obesity
10. Poor diet quality and pattern
11. Sedentary life-style

a recent study in *Medical World News,* a group of patients with fit life-styles was compared against a group whose life-styles were more typically sedentary and not fit. Over a 4-year period, there was a difference of more than $4,000 in costs of hospital and office expenses between these two groups. Today, our federal government is learning that the best way to contain health care costs involves long-range programs encouraging health and fitness as opposed to the previous illness- and crisis-oriented care.

Motivation

The motivation to adopt a positive life-style will arise from an understanding of the many positive benefits, not from scare tactics. Intelligent people who are told of their problems and the benefits that can result from a life-style change have the background to do three very important things. First, they can *understand* the need for change. One must know what is going on and why. Second, armed with this information, they can make a *commitment* to a life-style change. Third, taking this approach, emphasizing understanding and commitment, the change boils down very simply to a matter of *organization and scheduling.*

On selecting options for a life-style change (Table 2-2), I will not say much about cigarette smoking because it is self-explanatory. It simply has to stop. It is an extremely dangerous problem, essentially a premeditated suicide. The risks are not only pulmonary (cancer, emphysema, etc.), but the likelihood of hypertension, atherosclerosis, stroke, and heart attack are also increased. I believe it is also relevant for parents of small children to realize that their behavior influences their children's behavior. If they smoke, there is a greater chance their children will become smokers in later life. We also know that children who grow up with someone in the family smoking have a higher incidence of upper respiratory infections and allergies. If something a parent is doing technically harms a child, we have a

18

term for it: child abuse. If parents smoke in the presence of their children, they are guilty of potentially bringing harm to them.

Proper nutrition will be covered in detail in the next chapter. It suffices here to state that special calorie-counting or otherwise restricted diets (except for medical purposes) should be avoided. The quality and pattern of eating is enormously important. We are talking about permanent life-style changes rather than a short-term solution. If we eat a solid breakfast of high quality, a light lunch, and a moderate supper, we have gone a long way not only toward ensuring ourselves a better quality of performance during the day mentally and physically, but also toward supporting a good exercise program. I particularly emphasize eating large salads at supper because it is the problem meal in our society—much too large and full of too many things that have our metabolism struggling all night, thus making breakfast a much more difficult proposition. Eating a salad as the main or only dinner meal greatly reduces calories while providing excellent nutrition. Eating a good breakfast then becomes easier, as one is hungrier by morning.

From the preceding chapter you understand what aerobic fitness is and its benefits. You understand the misconception shared by much of society who wrongly view those who roll around with big muscles and are fairly trim as necessarily being in superb condition. Indeed, they may be isometrically in excellent condition, but the cardiovascular system may not have been well trained at all. It is not uncommon to find many of these weightlifters who are not aerobic exercisers in their forties and fifties either dead on arrival in the emergency room or staring in bewilderment at the coronary care unit ceiling after a heart attack.

There are many aerobic pursuits. Any activity that is nonintermittent and causes a relatively high heart rate qualifies. While cross-country skiing, roller skiing, and running rank at the top of the list in energy expenditure, the list is very long; in Chapter 4 I will discuss planning your own exercise prescription, taking into account particular likes, physical liabilities, time, and constraints. It is also important to attempt to undertake all of these changes simultaneously. You will often hear people say, "Let's see, this sounds like a lot. I would rather quit smoking and kind of wait on the other things, or maybe I'll do some exercise, but I'm not so sure about the diet or the smoking." I have found that if a person is going to make a life-style change and make a commitment to it, these activities support each other.

Safety should also be emphasized. A gradual progression is essential in any aerobic exercise program and particularly in jogging, which has the highest injury rate. I point out to people on a jogging-running program to concentrate on distance first, rather than worrying about pace. Too many people spend too much time thinking about what they did the day before or what their neighbor is doing. You must understand that this is your own individual program, and it is much more important to arrive at good distances safely and enjoyably than to go too hard too fast and invite injury.

Self-Reassessment and Reinforcement

Self-reassessment is an essential function if one is going to successfully achieve a life-style change. One cannot launch a boat, slide it into the water, break a bottle of champagne over it, and say good-bye and good luck. The boat still has to be steered and constant course corrections made if a successful voyage is to be made. To guard against the original motivation and excitement dwindling, interruptions occurring, and the life-style change going nowhere, you must carry out periodic self-assessments and make appropriate corrections.

I encourage you to keep a well-maintained exercise record. It should include a daily account of the type, duration, and intensity of primary exercise pursued. Any warm-up or cool-off exercises as well as the duration and type of any nonrecreational exercise (such as mowing the lawn, shoveling snow, or vacuuming the house) should also be listed.

Reinforcing one's progress is vital, as is praising all one is doing that is a step in the right direction, even if it is not quite up to the standards that have originally been outlined. Your record is your proof positive and a source of great self-satisfaction.

Chapter 3

Nutrition for Sports and Exercise

Food faddism may be more prominent in the area of athletics than in any other sphere of nutrition. Special dietary schemes to improve performance and endurance have been advocated by trainers, coaches, and athletes themselves since competitions first were held. The early Greek athletes consumed a vegetarian diet until 520 B.C., when Eurymenes of Samos decided that if animals ran fast so, too, might humans who ate their flesh. An overzealous disciple, Milo of Croton, is said to have consumed up to 20 pounds of meat a day.

More recent but equally invalid schemes include supplemental dietary wheat germ oil (a potent source of vitamin E and polyunsaturated fatty acids), gelatin (a source of glycine), phosphate, and alkalinizing agents. The practice of withholding a food such as milk because it causes "cotton mouth," curdles in the stomach, or lowers the respiratory quotient is equally fallacious. Perhaps in no area have more half-truths, myths, and just plain erroneous information been dispersed than in nutrition.

It goes without saying that a close relationship exists among diet, nutrition, and physical exercise. First, individuals who exercise regularly make heavy demands on their bodies' reserves of fluid and energy. One must be aware of the special dietary and nutritional needs created as a result of an exercise program. The ordinary diet will need to be supplemented and adjusted if one is to realize the maximum benefit from an exercise program. Before discussing the special dietary requirements of exercise, a few comments about general dietary objectives are appropriate.

The McGovern Committee, which recently studied American dietary habits, concluded that Americans eat too much and eat the wrong things. They consume too much meat, saturated fat, cholesterol, sugar, and salt. At the same time, they do not eat enough fruit, grain (especially whole

21

grain products), vegetables, and unsaturated fat. The committee urged American leaders to educate the public to increase its consumption of fruits, vegetables, and whole grain cereals and to sharply reduce its intake of fat and sugar.

Although new research constantly changes our perceptions about what we eat, the U.S. Dietary Goals still serve as informed guidelines for managing our diets. The goals include:

1. To avoid overweight, consume only as much energy (calories) as expended.

2. Increase complex carbohydrate consumption to about 48% of total calories.

3. Reduce overall fat consumption to 30% of calories.

4. Reduce saturated fat consumption and balance that with other fats.

5. Reduce cholesterol consumption to about 300 milligrams a day.

6. Reduce refined sugar consumption to about 10% of total calories.

7. Reduce salt consumption to 5 grams a day.

The suggestions of the committee, although physiologically sound, will not be easily implemented in this country. They run counter to long-standing ethnic and cultural eating patterns. Implementation may also cause heavy financial losses to major food producers and manufacturers who control food advertising, especially advertising of sugar-laden cereals that appeal to children. These companies may not welcome an attempt to change the financially successful "sugared" status quo.

Despite the expected resistance from cultural markets and big business, the recommended dietary changes will ultimately be realized. Today, Americans are more fitness conscious than ever before, and this enthusiasm will continue to increase. More Americans than ever before are engaging in strenuous physical exercise. Dietary lunacy is a necessary by-product of such concern for one's physical well-being. The old adage that you are what you eat is poignantly pertinent today.

Weight Loss Through Diet and Exercise

Body weight is lost when one or more of the body's substances is decreased, thus reducing total body mass. It is important to realize that a fundamental law of nature is that energy can neither be created nor destroyed, but its form can be changed—from mechanical to chemical to heat, for example. Fat is stored energy, and the body's fundamental energy equation is:

Calories consumed = calories used at rest by your body
+ calories used in exertion
+ calories stored as fat.

Weight loss is achieved when caloric intake is less than caloric expenditure. Short-term weight loss can be achieved by loss of water, fat, protein, or glycogen (a carbohydrate). Such weight loss occurs frequently during periods of strenuous exercise. Longer-term weight loss also depletes minerals from the bone and soft tissues of the body. Actually, weight loss is a simple biologic process that is related to the protein, glycogen, and water that exist in the body. Every gram of protein or glycogen has coupled with it approximately 3 to 4 grams of water. When a deficit of protein or glycogen occurs, there follows necessarily a water loss as well.

Until recently, it was thought that on the average, 1 pound (0.45 kg) of body weight loss corresponded to the burning of about 3500 kcal (kilocalories). This figure was derived from a value that suggested that 98% of the calories burned come from body fat. Studies now show that during the first several weeks of dietary restriction, weight loss far exceeds the caloric deficit and reflects primarily water loss. Much of this initial water loss is due to the increased urination that occurs with loss of sodium and water; water loss also occurs because the body's stores of glycogen are being depleted. Later in a caloric restriction diet, the water loss through increased urination (diuresis) stops entirely, and in some instances a water gain can occur while net losses of fat and protein continue.

It is of interest to note that different diets can produce an acceleration of weight loss due to greater water loss. For instance, a diet low in carbohydrates (the extreme being a fast) will cause a greater water diuresis and a quicker weight loss. During a prolonged caloric restriction (partial or total), the body gradually adapts by conserving protein and water and increasingly burning fat to make up the energy deficit. Studies show that obese individuals accomplish this adaptation more rapidly than lean people. However, the key finding is that the body's fat loss is essentially proportional to its energy deficit. So, in the end, the type of diet is relatively unimportant. What ultimately determines fat loss is the degree of caloric deprivation. Because of this, most nutritionists now recommend a balanced diet that combines smaller portions of the basic foods with a reduction or elimination of refined sugars and desserts. Such a diet not only accomplishes weight reduction, but also instills eating habits that help maintain the desired weight.

As surely as the sun rises and sets, there will always be one more diet that promises quick weight loss without effort. The latest fad is the "Last Chance Diet" or "Protein Supplemented Fasting," an essentially no-carbohydrate diet that supplies nutrition with a mixture of liquid proteins, vitamins, and minerals. The promoters of the Last Chance Diet claim that when protein is provided in the diet, the body does not use its own protein, thus minimizing muscle waste and the depletion of body protein stores. But is this really so? Not according to an article published in *The New England Journal of Medicine,* which recently reported, "Although some consider a low-calorie diet consisting entirely of protein to be uniquely advantageous in preserving body nitrogen, it has yet to be demonstrated convincingly that protein alone is more effective in this regard than an isocaloric mixture of protein and carbohydrate." Whenever carbohydrate intake is severely restricted, as it is in the Last Chance Diet, fat is mobilized, and rapid mobilization of fat may cause serious side effects including liver damage. Also, low potassium levels may result, and even cardiac arrhythmia deaths have been attributed to this diet. The chemical imbalance created by the loss of salt, water, and other minerals may lead to weakness, faintness, and other side effects. Even more tragic, because these diets do not encourage the proper way of eating, only one-third of those who follow them are able to keep fat off 18 months after abandoning them.

Influence of Diet and Exercise on Cholesterol, Cardiovascular Disease, and Atherosclerosis

The knowledge acquired over the past few decades about cholesterol, cardiovascular disease, and atherosclerosis (a kind of arteriosclerosis) indicates that a carefully combined program of diet and exercise can greatly retard these diseases. Arteriosclerosis is a process by which the walls of the blood vessels become infiltrated with fat, which in time calcifies and forms plaques that can occlude, or block, an artery. It is seldom localized. When it develops in a major vessel to the brain or lower extremities, for example, there is nearly always similar impairment of the coronary arteries. In fact, the major cause of death in patients following surgery for localized atherosclerosis is heart attack.

The precise mechanism by which cholesterol is deposited in the walls of arteries and an advanced plaque evolves is still being unraveled. It is apparent, though, that it involves a failure to properly metabolize cellular cholesterol as well as defects in smooth muscle cell proliferation. The means by which even normal cells are proliferated and build up cholesterol remain an enigma, but certain correlations regarding cholesterol are apparent.

Blood contains two classes of fats that are essential to life: cholesterol and triglycerides. Elevated levels of cholesterol or triglycerides or both are associated with accelerated atherosclerosis and an increased probability of heart attack. Of the many factors that influence the blood levels of these fats, diet, heredity, and exercise are the most important. Blood triglycerides and cholesterol can be reduced with exercise and with a diet low in saturated fats.

Cholesterol is transported by protein compounds called lipoproteins. Recent investigations have shown that the total level of cholesterol is of less importance than the ratio of high-density lipoprotein (HDL) to low-density lipoprotein (LDL). Low-density lipoproteins are the harmful transport vehicles that carry cholesterol into the tissues and enhance the buildup of fatty atherosclerotic plaques. Conversely, high-density lipoproteins are capable of transporting cholesterol out of arteries and tissues and into the liver, where it is broken down and eliminated. A high level of HDL to LDL correlates with a low risk for atherosclerosis and heart disease. Vigorous sustained exercise will raise high-density lipoprotein levels and lower low-density lipoprotein levels. A diet low in saturated fats will do the same. Triglycerides are also lowered by exercise and correlate with the HDL to

LDL ratio. Elevated triglyceride levels are seen with increased levels of low-density lipoprotein, while normal or low triglyceride levels are seen with high levels of high-density lipoprotein.

Is the Cholesterol Theory in Trouble?

Dr. George Mann of Vanderbilt University Medical School wrote: "A generation of research on the diet-heart question has ended in disarray. The official line since 1950 for management of the epidemic of coronary heart disease had been a dietary treatment. Foundations, scientists, and the media, both lay and scientific, have promoted low-fat, low-cholesterol poly-unsaturated diets, and the epidemic continues unabated, cholesterolemia in the population is unchanged, the clinicians are unconvinced of efficacy. . . . This litany of failures must lead the clinician to wonder where the proper research and solutions lie. The problem of coronary heart disease is real enough here, and yet it is rare in less developed societies. What aspect of life-style here makes atherosclerosis so malignant, its clinical consequences so fearsome?"

The cholesterol theory is traced back to 1808 to a Russian, I. A. Ignatovski, who was the first to demonstrate experimentally in rabbits that a high-protein, high-fat, high-cholesterol diet rapidly caused arteriosclerosis. His results were quickly confirmed, but his assumption that protein played a major role was never accepted. When Anitschkow and Chalatow in 1813 produced rapid arteriosclerosis in rabbits by feeding them high-cholesterol diets alone, the basic model that high dietary cholesterol causes athero-sclerosis was off and winging and has been popular ever since. It made no difference that others later showed that feeding rabbits high-protein diets with little or no cholesterol produced atherosclerosis even more rapidly; the cholesterol theory remained popular.

Why is the cholesterol theory being reevaluated in 1980? The answer lies in the fact that several very large and lengthy studies (one by the Mayo Clinic, another the Framingham Study sponsored by the National Institutes of Health) found little detectable relationship between diet cholesterol and serum cholesterol in people on a "normal" daily diet. This actually should not come as a great surprise, because cholesterol is not a foreign substance; most is synthesized by the body itself rather than derived from dietary sources. Our bodies will manufacture up to 1800 mg of cholesterol daily if none is eaten, and the amount our bodies produce drops as the amount we ingest increases. Thus, on a "normal" diet, it should come as no shock that whether one's cholesterol level is high or low depends on other factors, such as exercise, smoking, genetics, fiber in the diet, and so forth. Even more important when considering atherosclerosis is that while a diet that is low in cholesterol or that employs cholesterol lowering products (such as fiber and yogurt) may result in a 10 to 15% reduction in serum cholesterol, this may not be significant. The serum cholesterol levels of Americans are 100 to 200% above the New Guinean highlanders, in whom atherosclerosis is

Table 3-1
Cholesterol Level

Meat, Fish, Poultry, Eggs

(Average serving after cooking)	Cholesterol (mg)
Liver (3 oz, 85 g)	372
Egg (1 large, 50 g)	252
Shrimp, canned, drained solids (3 oz, 85 g)	128
Veal (3 oz, 85 g)	86
Lamb (3 oz, 85 g)	83
Beef (3 oz, 85 g)	80
Pork (3 oz, 85 g)	76
Chicken breast (½ breast, 80 g)	63
Lobster (3 oz, 85 g)	72
Clams, canned, drained solids (½ cup, 80 g)	50
Chicken drumstick (43 g)	39
Oysters, canned (3 oz, 85 g)	38
Fish, fillet (3 oz, 85 g)	34–75

Dairy Foods

Whole milk (8 oz, 244 g)	34
Cheddar & swiss cheese (1 oz, 28 g)	28
Ice cream (½ cup, 67 g)	27–49
American processed cheese (1 oz, 28 g)	25
Low fat (2%) milk (8 oz, 246 g)	22
Heavy whipping cream (1 tbsp, 15 g)	20
Yogurt, plain or vanilla (1 cup, 227 g)	17
Cream cheese (1 tbsp, 14 g)	16
Cottage cheese (½ cup, 134 g)	12–24
Butter (1 tsp, 5 g)	12
Sour cream (1 tbsp, 12 g)	8
Half-and-half (1 tbsp, 15 g)	6
Cottage cheese, dry curd (½ cup, 100 g)	6
Skim milk and buttermilk (8 oz, 245 g)	5

Desserts

Ladyfingers (4, 44 g)	157
Custard (½ cup, 133 g)	139
Apple pie (⅛ of 9″ pie, 114 g)	120
Custard pie (⅛ of 9″ pie, 114 g)	120
Lemon meringue pie (⅛ of 9″ pie, 105 g)	98
Bread pudding with raisins (½ cup, 133 g)	95
Peach pie (⅛ of 9″ pie, 114 g)	70
Pumpkin pie (⅛ of 9″ pie, 144 g)	70
Yellow cake, from mix (1/16 of 9″ cake, 75 g)	36
Chocolate cake, from mix (1/16 of 9″ cake, 69 g)	33
Brownie, homemade (1, 20 g)	17
Chocolate pudding, from mix (½ cup, 130 g)	15
Rice pudding with raisins (½ cup, 133 g)	15

rare. It is no wonder that the 10 to 15% reduction in serum cholesterol associated with even the strictest diets does not seem to make a major impact on the rate of atherosclerosis.

The milligrams of cholesterol contained in average servings of various foods are listed in Table 3-1.

Cholesterol, Homocysteine, Vitamin B₆, and Atherosclerosis

Currently, one of the most hotly contested scientific debates involves the homocysteine theory and the role of vitamin B_6 in the prevention of atherosclerosis. Homocysteine, a very toxic substance, is regularly produced from methionine, one of the amino acids that constitute all of the protein that we eat. Since the body does not manufacture methionine, it must be obtained from dietary sources. Normally, homocysteine is quickly converted to cystathionine, a nontoxic substance used in other biochemical reactions. A lack of vitamin B_6 leads to a reduction in conversion to cystathionine, a buildup of homocysteine in the blood, and the appearance of an oxidized form of homocysteine in the urine.

Kilmer McCully, a professor of pathology at Harvard Medical School, is generally credited with suggesting that homocysteine is the cause of atherosclerosis. He proposed in 1969 that too little vitamin B_6 would retard the conversion of homocysteine to cystathionine, lead to a buildup of homocysteine in the blood, and thus promote atherosclerosis. Implicit in this theory were several predictions as well as explanations for findings.

1. ·If homocysteine is maintained in the blood of experimental animals, atherosclerosis should develop.

2. Humans and experimental animals whose diets are deficient in vitamin B_6 should build up homocysteine in their blood.

3. People proven to have atherosclerosis, such as coronary patients, ought to show a tendency toward low vitamin B_6 in their blood.

In the last decade, each of these postulates has been found to be true, and thus the theory is gaining momentum. While a precise explanation of how homocysteine exerts its effects at the molecular level remains to be elucidated, the theory is alive and well, holding up nicely to its challenges.

Vitamin B_6 is plentiful in fruits and vegetables, less so in meats and dairy products. At a glance, it would seem unlikely that many people would be deficient in vitamin B_6. It must be realized, though, that 80 to 90% of vitamin B_6 is lost in milling wheat to white flour. Cooking vegetables inactivates two-thirds of their vitamin B_6, and cooking meat destroys 45% of the vitamin. Thus, it comes as no surprise that there are studies that show most Americans eating "normal" diets do not have adequate levels of vitamin B_6. This has been found to be the case especially in older Americans.

The homocysteine theory suggests most Americans eat too much protein and not enough vitamin B_6. It appears that a new criterion for selecting foods is on the horizon, based not just on cholesterol but on the relative B_6 and protein content (Table 3-2). While 2 mg per day of vitamin B_6 is

27

Table 3-2
Vitamin B$_6$ and Methionine Content of Some Foods

Food	B$_6$ (mg/100 g)	Methionine (mg/100 g)	B/M[a]
Apple (150 g)	.03	4	7.5
Avocado (123 g)	.42	19	22
Banana (150 g)	.51	11	46
Beans, raw, snap (1 c, 125 g)	.08	28	2.9
Beef, raw, round (3 oz, 85 g)	.50	970	0.5
Bread, white (1 slice, 23 g)	.04	126	0.3
Bread, whole wheat (1 slice, 23 g)	.18	161	1.1
Broccoli, raw (1 c, 150 g)	.19	54	3.6
Butter (1 tsp, 7 g)	.003	21	0.1
Carrots (50 g)	.15	10	15
Cheese, cheddar (1″ cube, 17 g)	.07	653	0.1
Chicken (½ breast, 76 g)	.5	537	0.9
Egg, hard-cooked (50 g)	.11	392	0.3
Lettuce (4″ head, 220 g)	.07	4	17
Milk, cow's, whole (1 c, 244 g)	.042	83	0.5
Oranges, raw (3″ diam., 210 g)	.06	2.7	22
Peanut butter (1 tbsp, 16 g)	.33	265	1.2
Peas, raw (1 c, 160 g)	.18	44	4.1
Potato, raw (100 g)	.25	25	10
Spinach, raw (180 g)	.28	54	5.2
Tomato, raw (150 g)	.10	8	12.5
Yogurt, plain (1 c, 246 g)	.032	102	0.3

[a] Ratio of B$_6$ to methionine ($\times 1000$).

currently an adequate amount, many Americans eat less than that, and there is considerable evidence to suggest that this level is too low to cover safely the entire adult population. Clearly, those groups prone to vitamin B$_6$ deficiency, such as pregnant and nursing mothers, women taking contraceptive pills, dieters (especially those on a high protein regimen), and elderly people, should receive more than 2 mg per day. Present evidence suggests that 10 mg per day of vitamin B$_6$ would provide a better margin of safety. Such a level would require a vitamin supplement, as it would not easily be found in our diet. But such levels are quite safe, because excessive vitamin B$_6$ is rapidly eliminated and the toxic dose of the vitamin is more than 1000 times 10 mg per day.

A great deal remains to be learned about homocysteine. Conclusive proof of the theory awaits not only a molecular understanding of its action on the cells of blood vessels, but also conclusive results from large-scale clinical testing over a number of years. Still, the cholesterol theory is

Table 3-3
U.S. Recommended Daily Allowances of Vitamins

Vitamin	Infants and children up to 4 years	Children 4 years to adult
Vitamin A	2500 IU	5000 IU
Thiamine (B_1)	0.7 mg	1.5 mg
Riboflavin (B_2)	0.8 mg	1.7 mg
Vitamin B_6	0.7 mg	2 mg
Vitamin B_{12}	3 mg	6 mg
Folacin (B_c)	0.2 mg	0.4 mg
Biotin	0.15 mg	0.3 mg
Niacin	9 mg	20 mg
Pantothenic acid	5 mg	10 mg
Ascorbic acid (C)	40 mg	60 mg
Vitamin D	400 IU	400 IU
Vitamin E	10 IU	30 IU

experiencing a renewed challenge and has been inadequate in explaining all aspects of atherosclerosis; thus, the homocysteine theory deserves serious consideration. It is suggested that a lower intake of protein and a higher amount of vitamin B_6 may be desirable.

Controversies Over Vitamins

For those following a strenuous daily exercise program, a knowledge of vitamins is absolutely essential, since there may be a special need for vitamin supplements to achieve maximum benefit from exercise.

No human, indeed no mammal, can be maintained on an exclusive diet of protein, carbohydrate, fat, and minerals. Additional factors present in natural foods are required in minute amounts (Table 3-3). These organic substances, vitamins, function as chemical regulators and are necessary for growth and the maintenance of life. There are 14 known vitamins and they are divided into two basic groups: those soluble in fat (vitamins A, D, E, and K) and those soluble in water (vitamin C and the B complex vitamins). Normally, a varied diet contains more than enough of these required vitamins. Because they do not contribute to body structure and are not a direct source of body energy, even the most active athlete needs little more than does the sedentary individual.

Since the advent of the industrial revolution and urbanization many people have not had access to a varied farm diet of recently harvested foodstuffs, and vitamin deficiencies have resulted. Sailors who spent months at sea without fruit or green vegetables developed scurvy from a lack of vitamin C. Impoverished Southeast Asians whose diets are restricted to polished rice develop vitamin B deficiencies, and infants in crowded European slums, deprived of adequate sunlight, develop rickets from a deficiency of vitamin D.

One man who has contributed much to our modern understanding of vitamin deficiency is Professor Victor Herbert. Professor Herbert states succinctly that "the sole unequivocal indication for vitamin therapy is vitamin deficiency."[9] He discusses six ways in which vitamin deficiency develops: inadequate ingestion, absorption, or utilization, and increased destruction, excretion, or requirement. Of the six possible causes of vitamin deficiency that Herbert cites, inadequate ingestion is the only indication for dietary vitamin supplementation.

The fat-soluble vitamins (A, D, E, and K) are stored in the liver and adipose tissue. Deficiencies develop only after months or years of inadequate intake, and excessive intake will cause abnormal accumulations and can produce toxic side effects. The water-soluble vitamins are not stored in the body and must be constantly replenished in the diet. Deficiencies can develop in weeks, and when excessive amounts are ingested, the excess is excreted in the urine, avoiding toxic accumulations.

Except during periods of extra nutrient demand, such as pregnancy, lactation, or prolonged illness, the American Medical Association does not recommend vitamin supplementation. Today, however, the use of multivitamin preparations is commonplace. This is not harmful so long as fat-soluble vitamins are not taken in excess. The essential foodstuffs can usually come from our diet and need not be found in any vitamin bottle. These "essential" nutrients—those that cannot be manufactured by the body—include water, sources of energy (primarily carbohydrates), nine amino acid building blocks of proteins, one fatty acid, a number of mineral elements, and vitamins. Only a diet including a selection from a wide variety of foods will ensure adequate essential nutrient intake.

Vitamins in Deficiency States

The AMA advised that the use of vitamin preparations as dietary supplements ought to be restricted to specific instances of deficiency; then, only the deficient vitamins in therapeutic amounts should be prescribed along with measures to correct any dietary inadequacies. Some common medical conditions requiring vitamin therapy include the malabsorption syndromes (tropical sprue and celiac disease), where vitamins A, D, E, and K may be required. Therapeutic amounts of folic acid or B_{12} or both are needed in specific deficiency states, including pernicious anemia. Pathologic conditions of the intestines that require bowel resection or intestinal bypass will require vitamin therapy, the specific needs being dictated by the location of the bowel resection. In burn victims and patients with extensive wounds to heal, vitamin C along with the B vitamins are frequently prescribed.

Thus, a number of specific deficiency states do require vitamin therapy.

To date, though, no conclusive evidence has been found to indicate that multivitamin preparations or megavitamin dosages have ever helped a patient. In fact, much critical research is immediately needed to be certain that no harmful effects are being sustained by such practices. The toxic effects of excessive intake of vitamins A and D and folic acid are known and, thus, the Food and Drug Administration restricts the amounts of these vitamins available over the counter. The question remains unanswered, however, regarding the possible harmful effects of prolonged megavitamin doses of any of the other vitamins.

The Vitamin C Controversy

No vitamin has aroused more controversy than vitamin C. This vitamin, which occurs naturally in citrus fruits such as oranges, lemons, and limes, was first recognized by James Lind, a physician in the eighteenth-century British Navy, who linked its deficiency with scurvy, the dreaded sailor's disease. During the era of the great sailing ships, sailors deprived of fresh fruit and vegetables for months on end developed scurvy, manifested by fatigue, easy bruising of the skin, and bleeding from the gums and mucous membranes. The scourge of the British Navy 200 years ago, this disease was greatly relieved by the discovery that fresh fruit, such as limes, would prevent it. The British sailors' use of limes earned them the nickname "Limeys." Although the protective value of limes was discovered in the 1700s, the specific protective agent in the lime was not identified as vitamin C until 1932.

Vitamin C is in the news again as the Nobel Prize-winning scientist Dr. Linus Pauling has proclaimed that large doses of vitamin C aid the body's defense mechanisms against infection. Controversy rages, but no conclusive proof exists that vitamin C in megadoses protects against the common cold or any other infection.

While the average nonexercising person may not need to supplement his diet with vitamin C, it has been shown that people who engage in high levels of physical stress or consume large quantities of alcohol deplete the body's stores of vitamin C. Smoking and even chewing tobacco (if the tobacco juice is swallowed) also lower vitamin C levels. Charcoal-broiled beef contains cholesterol oxide, a powerful oxidizer that quickly depletes both vitamins C and E. Our bodies cannot manufacture vitamin C; it must be ingested. Thus, it comes as no surprise that most athletes involved in endurance sports take 500 mg to 1 g of supplemental vitamin C per day.

A recent poll of members of the American Medical Joggers Association preparing for the Boston Marathon revealed that more than 90% of them took vitamin C as a supplement. While no scientific proof exists, many trainers and endurance athletes feel that supplemental vitamin C greatly reduces the incidence of muscle and tendon injuries. Vitamin C deficiency has also been implicated in the development of atherosclerosis. A deficiency of vitamin C may allow the lining of arteries (the endothelium) to degenerate and form sites for arteriosclerotic deposits.

From a medical standpoint, vitamin C supplements cause no harm, since excesses of vitamin C that the body cannot use are promptly excreted in the urine. Indeed, for the vigorously exercising individual, 500 mg to 1 g of vitamin C per day may well be beneficial. However, I must caution that ingestion of more than 4 g per day has been associated with kidney stones, so massive doses are distinctly discouraged.

Caffeine, Alcohol, and Physical Exercise

Presently there is considerable evidence to suggest that the ingestion of caffeine in the form of coffee, tea, or cola stimulates the sympathetic nervous system to mobilize free fatty acids (FFA). For endurance sports, such as long-distance running, this affords the competitor a slight advantage. For other than endurance sports, it is of no value.

Moderate to heavy coffee drinking was suggested to predispose to heart attack. More recent studies, however, show that coffee ingestion by itself is not harmful to the heart. These earlier reports failed to account for the fact that many coffee drinkers are also cigarette smokers, a practice that does predispose to heart attack, emphysema, and cancer. When cigarette smoking was taken into account, no increased incidence of heart attack was found in coffee drinkers.

Preliminary investigations have shown the rate of cancer of the pancreas to be two to three times higher in moderate to heavy coffee drinkers. The fact that no such correlation was found for tea suggests it is not caffeine per se that is the responsible agent. Since this was purely an epidemiological study, investigators are now attempting to confirm the initial findings.

Also contrary to earlier investigations, scientists now believe that moderate alcohol consumption is not harmful and indeed appears to protect the heart. Those who drank a "moderate" amount of beer had only half the incidence of heart attack as those who totally abstained. The mechanism appears to be a raising of the high-density lipoprotein-cholesterol (HDL-C) fraction. Both endurance exercise and moderate alcohol consumption raise HDL-C levels, which are known to protect against coronary heart disease. Marathoners who drank moderately had an even lower HDL-C than did fellow marathoners who abstained. This suggests that alcohol consumption is associated with an increase in HDL-C in excess of that resulting from vigorous exercise alone. The precise mechanism by which alcohol raises HDL-C levels is unknown.

Beer has long been a favorite thirst quencher for many distance runners, and it is now very popular as a replacement solution during the long-distance runs including marathons. Indeed, beer has been credited with keeping the kidneys functioning during endurance exercise by blocking antidiuretic hormone (ADH) secretion and thus preventing kidney stones and hematuria. It has a high potassium-to-sodium ratio (5:1) and, thus, is a safe sweat replacement preventing hypokalemia (potassium deficiency). It also replaces silicon and raises the level of high-density lipoproteins. While there is no proof that drinking beer will improve the performance of long-distance runners, it does appear that some discomfort may be alleviated.

One caution concerning alcohol consumption is its high caloric content of 7 calories per gram. Only fat, with 9 calories per gram, has more by comparison (protein and carbohydrates each contain only 4 calories per gram). Anyone who is dieting should be informed about the high caloric content of alcohol and avoid its use. All of us should be aware that excessive alcohol intake may cause direct toxic damage to the liver and in some cases to the heart as well. This is true even with an adequate diet. The old belief that cirrhosis of the liver develops primarily in people who drink heavily and eat poorly is myth, not fact. Today in the United States, it is estimated that there are more than 10 million alcoholics, and in urban areas cirrhosis of the liver is the third major cause of death between the ages of 25 and 65 years. Therefore, while moderate alcohol consumption, especially of beer, is certainly not harmful and may even protect the heart, heavy drinking is very hazardous and poisons the brain, heart, and liver. Recent investigations have prompted a warning from the Surgeon General that cancer has been linked to heavy alcohol consumption.

The Importance of Dietary Fiber
The most significant food sources of fiber are unprocessed wheat bran, unrefined breakfast cereals, and whole wheat and rye flours. Breads and cereals made from whole grain flours (wheat, rye, or oats) are highest in fiber, as are breakfast cereals with bran in the name. Additional sources include fresh and dried fruit, raw vegetables, and legumes. Those fruits with edible skin or seeds or both are highest in fiber. To obtain the highest fiber, the skin and pulp of the fruit should be eaten. It is not necessary to eat fruits and vegetables raw, because cooking does not affect fiber content. It appears that of all the sources, wheat bran is the most effective in increasing fecal bulk. This has led to commercial products of wheat bran on the grocery shelf with recommendations to add 6 teaspoons daily to everything from soup to chiffon cake.

Why is fiber important in our diet? Like many aspects of nutrition, there are known facts regarding fiber and other unproven speculations based on epidemiologic associations. First, let us review the hard data. Dietary fiber adds bulk to the diet. Because most sources are relatively low in calories, you feel full while you have consumed fewer calories than on a low-fiber diet. The increased bulk in your digestive tract greatly facilitates transit time. The average transit time is decreased from 48 hours to 12 hours when one switches from a low-fiber diet to a high-fiber diet.

A high-fiber diet also produces stools that are soft, more bulky, more frequent (average of one bowel movement every 19 hours), and contain twice as much carbohydrate, fat, and protein. More dietary fiber or "roughage" result in fecal nutrient loss that has been calculated to translate into energy losses that could account for an 8- to 10-lb weight difference over a 1-year period. Thus, a diet high in fiber aids in weight control or reduction in two ways: It not only allows one to feel full with fewer calories consumed, but also affords a greater fecal loss of calories. There is a double reduction in caloric uptake by the body.

A high-fiber diet also lowers blood cholesterol and especially low-density lipoprotein cholesterol levels. The precise mechanism by which dietary fiber lowers cholesterol is unknown; the fact that it occurs, however, raises speculation that the amount of fiber in the diet may be a factor in the prevention of atherosclerosis.

The intake of crude fiber in the American diet has dropped by about one-third since the turn of the century. While the intake of fiber from vegetables has remained relatively constant, that from potatoes, fruit, cereals, dry peas, and beans has declined. Coincident with this reduction of dietary fiber has been an increase in a host of ailments including coronary heart disease, cholesterol gallstones, diabetes, obesity, hiatal hernia, peptic ulcer, constipation, diverticulosis, hemorrhoids, varicose veins, and cancer of the colon. All of these have been linked to overconsumption of sucrose and highly milled starches, and underconsumption of fibrous materials in the diet. While most of the postulates remain controversial and inconclusive and are based on epidemiologic relationships (that is, populations in the world with high-fiber diets who have a low incidence of these problems), it is still interesting to recapitulate the physiologic explanation.

Fiber, by adding bulk to the feces, will eliminate constipation and in over 70% of people render diverticulosis asymptomatic. To the extent the stool is soft and one does not have to strain, the problem of hemorrhoids is lessened. Obesity can be combated by a high-fiber diet as previously discussed, and its control affords a reduction in adult-onset diabetes and problems of varicosities. The anti-obesity and cholesterol-lowering effect of fiber are both cited to explain its beneficial effect on heart disease. The cholesterol-lowering effects account for the alleviation of cholesterol gallstones.

The transit time of feces may be a factor in hiatal hernia, ulcer, and, most important, colon cancer. In the last half century, while the fiber consumption from fruits and vegetables has decreased by 20% and that from cereals and grains 50%, the incidence of colon cancer has risen significantly. It has been speculated that by decreasing the transit time through the colon by one-third of the carcinogen or cancer provoking agent, be it a virus or food breakdown product, the carcinogen is exposed to the large bowel for a much shorter period of time. It, therefore, has a diminished opportunity to break down the natural resistance of the colon and produce cancer.

Whether fiber is of any benefit in preventing colon cancer or not, most Americans do need to increase the fiber content of their diets to achieve the

Table 3-4
High-Fiber Foods

	Serving Size	Amount Fiber
Apple	3.5 oz	1.0 g
Apricots	3.5 oz	3.0 g
Beans (green)	3.5 oz	1.1 g
Boysenberries	3.5 oz	1.8 g
Bran breakfast cereals (e.g., Kellogg's *Bran Buds*)	1 oz (⅓ cup)	8.0 g
Quaker Oats	1 oz (⅓ cup)	.3 g
Bread (whole wheat)	2 slices	.8 g
Cauliflower	3.5 oz	1.0 g
Corn	6 oz	.44 g
Cucumber	3.5 oz	.6 g
Eggplant	3.5 oz	.9 g
Macedonia nuts	3.5 oz	1.25 g
Pears	3.5 oz	1.4 g
Rice	⅓ cup	.5 g
Strawberries	3.t oz	.8 g
Sunflower seeds	3.5 oz	1.25 g
Tomatoes	3.5 oz	.5 g

known beneficial effects just discussed. Table 3-4 lists foods especially high in fiber. While some may wish to sprinkle bran on various foods or substitute one-fifth bran for an equal part of flour in any baked items from cakes to waffles, for most of us a significant increase in dietary fiber is achieved by enjoying unprocessed cereals, a slice of whole wheat bread, a salad, and some fresh or processed fruit on a regular basis.

Nutrition for Endurance Sports

The primary dietary requirements for the endurance athlete are increased caloric intake plus increased fluid consumption, each equal to their respective losses. The vitamin, mineral, and protein needs of most athletes are little different from sedentary spectators. Energy is provided very inefficiently by protein; better by fats, which should be largely polyunsaturated; and best by carbohydrates. This means the food servings should be larger, particularly in carbohydrates such as cereals, grains, and the natural sugars found in fruit. Except for endurance sports, the diet matters little to performance. To understand why increased carbohydrates are important to endurance performance, it is helpful to review the metabolism of exercise.

The Metabolism of Exercise

While fat and carbohydrate each contribute about 40% of the caloric content of the average American or European diet, the body stores fuel almost entirely (80 to 85%) in the form of fat (FFA stores in adipose tissue). The remainder of our immediate fuel stores is glucose stored in our muscles and the liver as glycogen. During the earliest phase of muscular activity— the first 5 to 10 minutes—glucose stored in the muscles is the major fuel source. By consuming a diet high in carbohydrates for 48 to 72 hours prior to vigorous prolonged competition, a "muscle glycogen super compensation" can be achieved. This "overloading" of muscle glycogen is further enhanced if the muscles are first exercised to the point of glycogen depletion (exhaustion). Only in those muscles exercised does this glycogen over-storage occur. This practice, called "carbohydrate loading," thus affords the exercising muscle a greater initial store of energy. Therefore, in the three or four days preceding endurance competition, the diet should be shifted to 75 to 90% carbohydrates to ensure the "muscle glycogen super compensation."

As exercise continues, glucose is released from the liver, and muscle blood flow and glucose uptake rises to 7 to 20 times the resting level, depending on the intensity of the exercise performed. Initially most of the glucose released from the liver is from glycogenolysis, the release of glucose already stored in the liver as glycogen. The glycogen stores in the liver are also enhanced by a diet high in carbohydrates. As the duration and intensity of exercise increases, a greater amount of liver glucose release occurs from the process of gluconeogenesis. Gluconeogenesis, which is the synthesis or manufacture of glucose from its substrate precursors (lactate, pyruvate, glycerol, and amino acids), increases from about 10% at rest to more than 40% of hepatic glucose release after 4 hours of exercise.

After 40 minutes of exercise, blood-born glucose is responsible for 70 to 90% of the glucose metabolized. However, in prolonged exercise, between 1 and 4 hours, the blood glucose level falls progressively, and the level of free fatty acids released from adipose tissue rises to become the major fuel source. A slight fall in blood glucose occurs because the hepatic glucose output fails to keep pace with the greatly augmented increase in muscle uptake and use of glucose. Thus, there are three phases of fuel use in prolonged exercise. First, the muscle burns glucose already stored in it; then, glucose, primarily released from the liver, is taken from the blood stream; and finally, the main fuel source is free fatty acids from the body's fat stores. Endurance exercise enhances the body's ability to mobilize and metabolize free fatty acids.

After exercise ceases, the blood flow to muscles decreases, but the uptake of glucose remains three to four times the resting level for nearly an hour. The full replenishment of muscle glycogen takes about 48 hours to be complete. Liver glycogen replenishment, on the other hand, is complete in 24 hours. Insulin levels rise after exercise to facilitate this response. How-

36

ever, *during exercise, insulin levels decrease, yet muscle uptake of glucose is enhanced.* This indicates that the muscle uptake of glucose during exercise does not require increased insulin. The exact mechanism by which exercising muscle can take glucose from the blood stream and use it is not fully understood. Endurance training enhances this process so that insulin sensitivity is enhanced, a lesser amount facilitating a greater muscle glucose uptake.

The Ideal Precompetition Meal

The pre-exercise meal contributes little to the energy requirements of the impending event, since it requires up to 24 hours to restore liver glycogen and 48 hours to replenish muscle glycogen. The precompetition meal should serve the following needs: minimize hunger, ensure hydration equal to expected fluid losses, provide for prompt emptying of the gastro-intestinal tract, protect against nausea, and, to a degree, reflect individual food preferences.

Fluid losses, of course, will depend on air temperatures and on the intensity and duration of exercise. While fluid should be replaced during vigorous exercise, it should be realized that the intestinal tract absorbs water at about 60 ml per hour. Thus, if you are perspiring freely, you cannot keep up with the water loss simply by drinking fluids. For this reason, endurance athletes such as marathon runners, who know they will lose 4 to 8 pounds of water during a given marathon, spend the hours immediately before the race drinking fluids until their urine is clear. They actually start the race with several extra pounds of water in their bodies that will quickly be lost as the race unfolds. Likewise, the vigorously exercising adult should precede his or her workout by drinking fluids. Remember that thirst is not immediately sensitive to serious body dehydration. Thus, plan your increased fluid consumption based on anticipated fluid losses.

Too much has been made of the fact that we lose salt when we perspire. Actually, well-conditioned athletes lose only trace amounts of salt in their sweat, and their kidneys become proficient at losing very little sodium in the urine. Habitual exercisers should not be concerned about salt needs, as long as their diets are well rounded. Salt is ubiquitous in processed foods and already overly plentiful in most diets. For most people, three daily meals easily replace the salt lost in up to 10 pounds of exercise-induced sweat. Thus, there is no need to reach for the salt shaker during the precompetition meal.

The precompetition meal should be light (approximately 500 calories), consist mainly of carbohydrate, and be consumed 3 to 4 hours before the event. Carbohydrates rapidly empty from the stomach and do not produce diuresis. The practice of taking sugar or honey for a "quick energy lift" a half hour before the event actually impairs performance. This is because the rapid rise in blood glucose causes the release of extra insulin, which in turn impairs the release and muscle use of free fatty acids. This places greater energy requirements on muscle glycogen and blood glucose and can result in hypoglycemia after the exercise begins. Performance can be impaired by as much as 19%.

A heavy meal, especially one containing sizable portions of fat and protein, consumed within two hours of competition also impairs performance. Thus, the traditional pregame steak dinner is not recommended as a desirable nutritional preparation for vigorous exercise. Protein, a virtually useless source of immediate energy, compromises hydration by increasing urine. Fat delays emptying of the stomach and upper gastrointestinal tract, thereby impairing respiration and placing excessive stress on the circulation. This can also lead to nausea and vomiting.

In the two hours immediately before the event, it is best to consume no solid foods, but clear fluids of low caloric content may be consumed in limited amounts. Caffeine has been shown to mobilize FFA and, thus, make more fat available for energy. For this reason, many endurance athletes will drink a cup or two of a caffeine drink (coffee, tea, cola) shortly before the event. Once exercise has commenced, the ingestion of sugar does not cause a rise in plasma insulin. Sugar taken during exercise tends to maintain blood glucose levels and retard the breakdown of liver glycogen. It is presently unproven, however, whether glucose taken during competition enhances performance.

Chapter 4

Your Personal Aerobic Exercise Prescription

Determining Your Level of Fitness

Before you begin an exercise program, you should undergo a thorough physical examination. It should include a family history of relevant medical problems and familial traits, a blood lipid profile, resting blood pressure, and a resting 12-lead electrocardiogram (EKG). If you are over 35 and have not been regularly exercising, an exercise 12-lead EKG is also recommended. It is by stressing the heart in this manner that irregular heartbeats and signs of heart strain can best be detected. If heart irregularities appear, your exercise program may have to be greatly modified to avoid the risk of heart attack. Gradually, as your stress EKG improves, your level of physical conditioning can be advanced.

The stress electrocardiogram is especially important for one who has previously been sedentary and had little regular exercise or who has a family history of heart disease. The test is not necessary in one who already engages in daily aerobic exercise. Your maximal heart rate—that rate of exertion that leaves you totally out of breath—and associated blood pressure should also be recorded.

Finally, it is helpful, although not essential, to have your maximum oxygen uptake recorded. Many community hospitals and virtually all large teaching medical centers carry out this test. It permits an objective comparison of your present level of fitness with age-related tables, giving an accurate indication of not only your present fitness, but also your performance capability. By repeating the examination at specific intervals after beginning an exercise program, your rate of fitness improvement can be documented. Obviously, such a test is immensely useful to coaches and competitive athletes planning training programs.

Figure 4–1

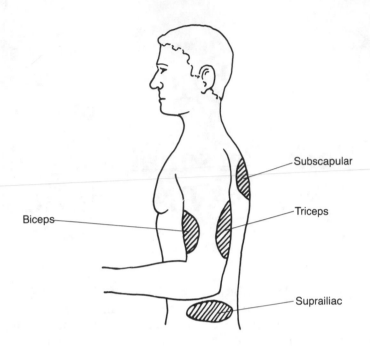

Although a test of maximal oxygen consumption (VO_2 max) is the most precise measurement of one's fitness, practical considerations make this test undesirable for all but the superbly conditioned athlete. Since the endpoint is exhaustion, one must consider whether the subject quit short of exhaustion because of low tolerance to physical discomfort, lack of motivation, or even fear of a coronary.

Because of these drawbacks, *submaximal oxygen consumption testing* is the test most used to determine fitness. It is based on the fact that oxygen consumption and heart rate both increase in a straight line in response to increased physical effort. Thus, this test involves physical effort, usually either running on a treadmill or riding a bicycle ergometer, that brings the heart rate up approximately to 50% and then to 75% of one's age-computed maximal level as read from tables. Your oxygen consumption is measured at these two levels, and from them your maximal VO_2 max is calculated. There is also a simplification of the submaximal test that uses tables to relate heart rate and oxygen consumption. Here, heart rate is plotted against work load to obtain a predicted VO_2 max from a table of average equivalents. This is accurate within a range of 10% and eliminates the need to collect and analyze expired air and, thus, becomes practical in an office setting.

Although not essential, your complete fitness exam should include an assessment of body composition, or lean body mass versus body fat. The only precise method of determining body fat is the immersion technique, but this is unavailable except in certain exercise laboratories. However, an adequate alternative technique you can perform on yourself involves measuring your body fat at four sites: behind the triceps muscles (back of the upper arm), over the biceps muscle (front of upper arm), at the inferior angle of the scapula (shoulder blade), and the suprailiac (vertical skin fold on the crest of the hip) (see Figure 4-1). Use a caliper to measure the skin fold thickness in each area in millimeters, and then add up the total millimeters: This is your fat index. Table 4-1 allows you to compute your percentage of body fat ($\pm 5\%$) and gives suggested percents at various ages. Repeat these measurements as your fitness schedule progresses. You can anticipate a 20 to 25% reduction in skin-fold fat measurements, even if you have not lost any total body weight. If dieting is used in conjunction with exercise, a much greater reduction of body fat will occur.

Since muscle weighs more than fat, it is possible to sustain a given weight during an exercise program and still lose considerable body fat. This is especially true for the already lean person. Those underweight may even experience a slight weight gain as muscle is added. This principle applies to the conditioning of the cardiovascular-pulmonary system.

Table 4-1
Fat Content, as Percentage of Body Weight,
for the Sum of Four Skin Folds

Skin Folds, mm	Males (age in years)				Females (age in years)			
	17-29	30–39	40–49	50+	16–29	30–39	40–49	50+
15	4.8	—	—	—	10.5	—	—	—
20	8.1	12.2	12.2	12.6	14.1	17.0	19.8	21.4
25	10.5	14.2	15.0	15.6	16.8	19.4	22.2	24.0
30	12.9	16.2	17.7	18.6	19.5	21.8	24.5	26.6
35	14.7	17.7	19.6	20.8	21.5	23.7	26.4	28.5
40	16.4	19.2	21.4	22.0	28.4	25.5	28.2	30.3
45	17.7	20.4	23.0	24.7	25.0	26.9	29.6	31.9
50	19.0	21.5	24.6	26.5	26.5	28.2	31.0	33.4
55	20.1	22.5	25.9	27.9	27.8	29.4	32.1	34.6
60	21.2	23.5	27.1	29.2	29.1	30.6	33.2	35.7
65	22.2	24.3	28.2	30.4	30.2	31.6	34.1	36.7
70	23.1	25.1	29.3	31.6	31.2	32.5	35.0	37.7
75	24.0	25.9	30.3	32.7	32.2	33.4	35.9	38.7
80	24.8	26.6	31.2	33.8	35.1	34.3	36.7	39.6
85	25.8	27.2	32.1	34.8	34.0	35.1	37.5	40.4

Table 4-1 (continued)
Fat Content, as Percentage of Body Weight,
for the Sum of Four Skin Folds

Skin Folds, mm	Males (age in years)				Females (age in years)			
	17-29	30–39	40–49	50+	16–29	30–39	40–49	50+
90	26.2	27.8	33.0	35.8	34.8	35.8	38.3	41.2
95	26.9	28.4	33.7	36.6	35.6	36.5	39.0	41.9
100	27.6	29.0	34.4	37.4	36.4	37.2	39.7	42.6
105	28.2	29.6	35.1	38.2	37.1	37.9	40.4	43.3
110	28.8	30.1	35.8	39.0	37.8	38.6	41.0	43.9
115	29.4	30.6	36.4	39.7	38.4	39.1	41.5	44.5
120	30.0	31.1	37.0	40.4	39.0	39.6	42.0	45.1
125	30.5	31.5	37.6	41.1	39.6	40.1	42.5	45.7
130	31.0	31.9	38.2	41.8	40.2	40.6	43.0	46.2
135	31.5	32.3	38.7	42.4	40.8	41.1	43.5	46.7
140	32.0	32.7	39.2	43.0	41.3	41.6	44.0	47.2
145	32.5	33.1	39.7	43.6	41.8	42.1	44.5	47.7
150	32.9	33.5	40.2	44.1	42.3	42.6	45.0	48.2
155	33.3	33.9	40.7	44.6	42.8	43.1	45.4	48.7
160	33.7	34.3	41.2	45.1	43.3	43.6	45.8	49.2
165	34.1	34.6	41.6	45.6	43.7	44.0	46.2	49.6
170	34.5	34.8	42.0	46.1	44.1	44.4	46.6	50.0
Maximum Desirable Percentage	12.0	20.0	22.0	25.0	23.0	27.0	30.0	34.0

Finally, to increase the efficiency of the heart and lungs, it is essential to perform continuous rhythmic exercises long enough to stress the cardio-vascular-pulmonary system. Thus, brisk walking, jogging, bicycling, or cross-country skiing should be maintained until the body begins to perspire and the pulse rate rises above 130 beats per minute for several minutes. Within 10 minutes after exertion, your pulse rate should return to normal and you should not feel fatigued. If the return to normal does not occur, you are advancing too fast.

Finding Your Fitness Level

Although I urge you to see a qualified physician to receive a fitness examination and a subsequent exercise prescription, I know not all of you will or can comply. Before you proceed with the tests and programs described in the rest of this chapter, let me reiterate my recommendation that you first obtain a fitness examination and commence the program under a qualified physician's supervision.

Table 4-2
Energy Expenditures for Heavy Activities

Recreational Activities
(600–900 calories burned/hour)

Bicycling (10 mph uphill)*	Mountain climbing
Cross-country skiing	Roller skiing
Deep-sea fishing (with fish on)*	Rugby
Handball	Swimming*
Jogging†	

Household Activities
(7–10 calories per minute for a 150-pound person.
To be used as an endurance workout, these activities must be pursued
very vigorously in a nonstop manner for 30–45 minutes.)

Chopping wood	Shoveling dirt, sand, manure, etc.
Digging holes	Carrying anything over 50 pounds
Shoveling snow	Moderate activities done vigorously so
Walking up steep hills	as to produce a heart rate of 120–130
Walking up stairs	beats per minute.
Carrying 30–50 pounds up an incline	

*Recommended for persons over 50 by the International Committee for the Standardization of Physical Fitness
†Should be approached cautiously by those with back problems.
**From *Diabetes and Exercise* by Robert C. Cantu, M.D., F.A.C.S. Copyright © by Robert C. Cantu. Reprinted by permission of the publisher, E. P. Dutton, Inc.

You can determine your own level of fitness by simple tests. The walk test is the easiest. The intent of the walk test is to determine how many minutes, up to a total of 10, you can walk briskly on a flat surface without experiencing undue shortness of breath or discomfort. If you can walk briskly for only 3 minutes or less, you are at Level 3, the Basic Level. If you can easily exceed 3 minutes but cannot comfortably walk 10 minutes, you are at Level 2, or Moderate Fitness. If you can easily walk 10 minutes, then you may be at Level 1. To determine if you are at Level 1, an additional test can be attempted; it consists of walking and jogging. Alternately walk 50 steps and jog 50 steps for a total of 6 minutes. Walk at a rate of at least 120 steps per minute and jog at a rate of 144 steps per minute. If you must stop this test before 6 minutes have elapsed, you are at Level 2. If you can easily complete the 6-minute test, you are at Level 1. If you can complete 12 minutes of this test, you can move beyond Level 1 to any of the endurance sports (jogging, swimming, cycling, and cross-country skiing) (see Table 4-2).

To be of maximum value, your exercises should be done three to four times a week. A half-hour should be sufficient time. Start easily and slowly and increase the tempo and number of repetitions. If you feel a little stiff, do not let this deter you. However, if you experience actual pain that does not disappear within 48 hours, don't use that exercise until medical clearance is given and the exercise can be resumed without pain. The exercises for each level(1, 2, and 3) should be carried out in the sequence given, because both a warm-up and a cooling-off period are built into each series. The cooling-off period has recently received much attention in the Olympic games. It has been shown that the cooling-off phase allows muscles to be drained of lactic acids, the products of aerobic metabolism, and it is the best way to prepare the body for the next day's strenuous activity. If possible, keep a log or record of the exercises you perform, how many repetitions you do, and how much time you require. Many find that doing the exercises to music makes them more enjoyable. Others find that watching TV or listening to the radio while exercising relieves boredom. The exercises can be done alone or with family or friends. Clothing should be loose, comfortable, and stretchable, not restrictive. Shoes should have no heels and nonskid soles.

Your Own Exercise Program Based on Your Level of Fitness

Level 3: The Basic Level
You should attempt to complete the entire sequence of exercises in Level 3 without rest periods of more than 2 minutes. If necessary, however, as you begin, take a longer rest period, but try to finish the entire sequence. An indication of improvement in your level of fitness will be your ability to complete the sequence comfortably in less time. Never execute an exercise in a jerky manner to increase speed. All exercises should be done as smoothly and comfortably as possible.
1. Walk; 3 minutes (Exercise 1)
2. Bend and Stretch; 2 repetitions increasing to 10 repetitions (Exercise 3)
3. Rotate head; 2 increasing to 10 repetitions each way (Exercise 4)
4. Body Bender; 2 increasing to 5 repetitions (Exercise 5)
5. Back Flattener; 2 increasing to 5 repetitions (Exercise 6)
6. Wall Press; 2 increasing to 5 repetitions (Exercise 7)
7. Arm Circles; 5 repetitions each way (Exercise 9)
8. Wing stretcher; 2 increasing to 5 repetitions (Exercise 11)
9. Single Knee Raise; 3 increasing to 10 repetitions (Exercise 13)
10. Straight Arm and Leg Stretch; 2 increasing to 5 repetitions (Exercise 18)
11. Heel-Toe Walk (Exercise 19)
12. Side Leg Raise; 2 increasing to 5 repetitions each leg (Exercise 23)
13. Partial Sit-up; 2 increasing to 10 repetitions (Exercise 24)
14. Alternate Walk-Jog; 1 to 3 minutes (Exercise 2)
15. Walk; 1 to 3 minutes (Exercise 1)

For the first week do the fewest repetitions or shortest duration of time shown for each exercise. If after a week you still find that this level requires a strenuous effort, do not increase the duration or repetitions. Only when you feel comfortable with an exercise where a range of repetitions is given should you slowly increase the number by one additional repetition per week. When you can carry out the maximum number of repetitions indicated for each exercise without resting between, you are ready to move on to Level 2.

Level 2: Moderate Fitness

For the Level 2 exercise program, you should proceed in a manner similar to Level 3. Start with the fewest number of repetitions and gradually advance one repetition at a time until you are capable of performing the highest continuous number of repetitions of each exercise. When this can be accomplished without straining or undue fatigue, you are ready to advance to Level 1.

1. Walk; 3 minutes (Exercise 1)
2. Bend and Stretch; 10 repetitions (Exercise 3)
3. RotateHead; 10 repetitions each way (Exercise 4)
4. Body Bender; 5 increasing to 10 repetitions (Exercise 5)
5. Back Flattener; 5 increasing to 10 repetitions (Exercise 6)
6. Wall Press; 5 repetitions (Exercise 7)
7. Arm Circles; 5 increasing to 10 repetitions (Exercise 9)
8. Half-Knee Bend; 5 increasing to 10 repetitions (Exercise 10)
9. Wing Stretcher; 5 increasing to 10 repetitions (Exercise 11)
10. Single Knee Hug; 3 increasing to 10 repetitions (Exercise 14)
11. Single Leg Raise; 3 increasing to 10 repetitions (Exercise 16)
12. Straight Arm and Leg Stretch; 5 repetitions (Exercise 18)
13. Heel-Toe Beam Walk (Exercise 20)
14. Knee Push-up; 2 increasing to 10 repetitions (Exercise 22)
15. Side Leg Raise; 2 increasing to 10 repetitions each leg (Exercise 23)
16. Advanced Sit-up; 2 increasing to 10 repetitions each leg (Exercise 25)
17. Sitting Bend; 2 increasing to 5 repetitions (Exercise 27)
18. Deep Knee Bend; 2 increasing to 5 repetitions (Exercise 29)
19. Alternate Walk-Jog; 3 increasing to 6 minutes (Exercise 2)
20. Walk; 1 increasing to 3 minutes (Exercise 1)

Level 1: Good Fitness

The same directions, starting with the fewest repetitions and gradually increasing, apply for Level 1. When you can perform the maximum repetitions without rest periods, you can either continue to increase the number of repetitions and speed of their execution or advance to other more vigorous exercises and sports as discussed in Chapter 8.

1. Alternately walk 50 steps and jog 50 steps for 3 minutes (Exercise 2)

2. Bend and Stretch; 10 repetitions (Exercise 3)
3. Rotate Head; 10 repetitions each way (Exercise 4)
4. Body Bender; 10 repetitions (Exercise 5)
5. Back Flattener with legs extended; 10 repetitions (Exercise 6)
5. Wall Press; 5 repetitions (Exercise 7)
7. Posture Check; 5 repetitions (Exercise 8)
8. Arm Circles; 10 increasing to 15 repetitions each way (Exercise 9)
9. Half Knee Bend; 10 increasing to 20 repetitions (Exercise 10)
10. Wing Stretcher; 10 increasing to 20 repetitions (Exercise 11)
11. Wall Push-up; 10 repetitions (Exercise 12)
12. Double Knee Hug; 3 increasing to 10 repetitions (Exercise 15)
13. Single Leg Raise and Knee Hug; 3 increasing to 10 repetitions (Exercise 17)
14. Straight Arm and Leg Stretch; 5 repetitions (Exercise 18)
15. Heel-Toe Beam Walk (Exercise 20)
16. Hop; 5 repetitions on each foot (Exercise 21)
17. Knee Push-up; 5 increasing to 10 repetitions (Exercise 22)
18. Side Leg Raise; 10 repetitions each leg (Exercise 23)
19. Advanced Modified Situp; 2 increasing to 10 repetitions (Exercise 26)
20. Sitting Bend; 5 increasing to 10 repetitions (Exercise 27)
21. Diver's Stance; hold 10 seconds (Exercise 28)
22. Deep Knee Bends; 5 increasing to 10 repetitions (Exercise 29)
23. Alternate Walk-Jog; 5 minutes (exercise 2)
24. Walk; 3 minutes (Exercise 1)

Exercises Used in All Three Basic Levels

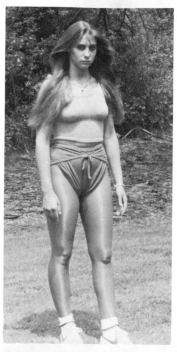

Exercise 1. Walk (3 Minutes)

Objective: An excellent warm-up exercise to loosen muscles and prepare you for the ensuing exercises.

Basic Exercise: Stand erect and be well balanced on the balls of your feet. Begin walking rapidly on a level surface.

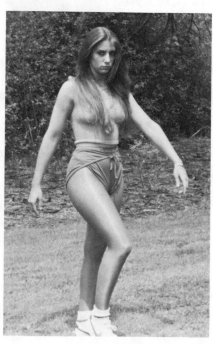

Exercise 2. Alternate Walk-Jog
(3 Minutes)

Objective: Warm-up exercise for more advanced exercises; good for legs and circulation.

Basic Exercise: Stand erect, as for walking, with arms held flexed and forearms roughly parallel to the floor. Begin walking for 50 steps, then break into a slow run (jog) for 50 steps. When jogging, stride easily, landing on your heels and rolling to push off on your toes. This heel-toe movement is in contrast to a fast run where you land and stay on the balls of your feet. Arms should swing freely from the shoulders in opposition to the legs. Breathing should be deep, but never labored to the point of gasping. Continue for 3 minutes.

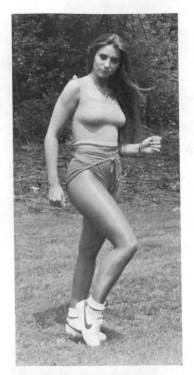

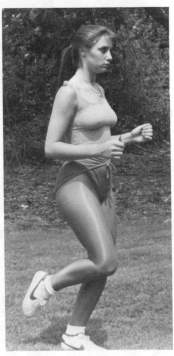

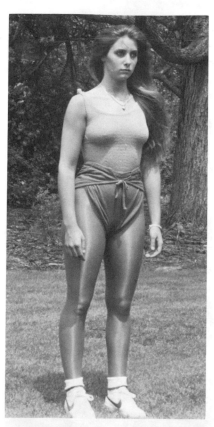

Exercise 3. Bend and Stretch

Objective: To loosen and stretch primarily the back, hamstring, and calf muscles.

Basic Exercise: Stand erect, with your feet shoulder-width apart. Slowly bend forward at the waist and touch your outstretched fingers to your toes, bending your knees to whatever degree is necessary to accomplish this maneuver. The maximal effort is achieved when the knees can remain locked. Return slowly and smoothly to the starting position.

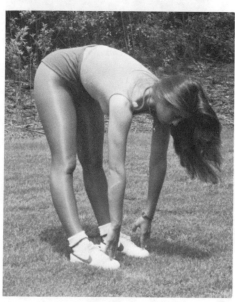

Exercise 4. Rotate Head

Objective: To loosen and relax the muscles of the neck and to firm up the throat and chin line.

Basic Exercise: Stand erect, with your feet shoulder-width apart and your hands on your hips. Slowly, in a smooth motion, rotate your head in a full circle, stretching from left to right; then slowly rotate your head in a full circle stretching from right to left.

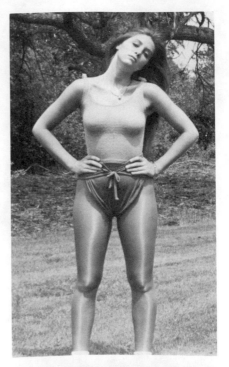

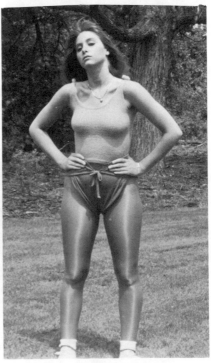

50

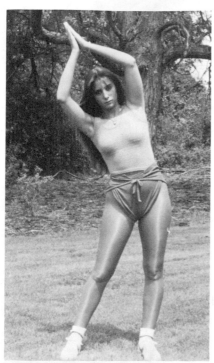

Exercise 5. Body Bender

Objective: To stretch arm, trunk, and leg muscles.

Basic Exercise: Stand erect, with your feet shoulder-width apart and your hands extended overhead with your palms together. Bend at the waist, stretching gently and slowly sideward to the left as far as possible while keeping your hands together and your arms extended straight; return to starting position; repeat same movements to the right.

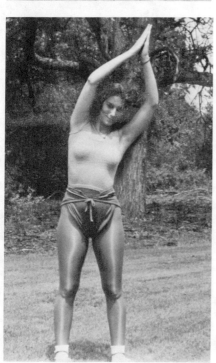

Exercise 6. Back Flattener

Objective: To strengthen gluteal (buttock) and abdominal muscles and flatten the lower back.

Basic Exercise: Lie on your back on padded floor with knees well bend. Relax with arms above your head. You may place a small pillow under your head. Now squeeze your buttocks together as if trying to hold a piece of paper between them. At the same time suck in and tighten the muscles of your abdomen. You should feel your back flatten against the floor. This is the *flat back position.* Hold this position for a count of 10 (10 seconds); relax and then repeat the exercise three times in the beginning. Gradually attempt to increase to 20 repetitions.

Advanced Modifications:

Buttock Raise: After the basic exercise has been done for a week or more, additional flattening can be achieved by doing the exercise with the buttocks slightly raised off the floor (1 to 2 inches) at the time the buttocks are squeezed and the abdomen tensed. Hold for the count of 10; relax and repeat.

Legs Extended: After several weeks of the basic exercise, gradually do the exercise with the knees less and less bent until you can execute the exercise with your legs straight. The buttock raise need not be combined with this modification.

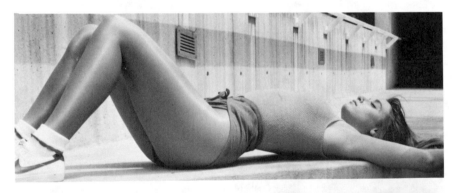

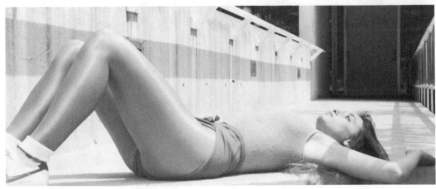

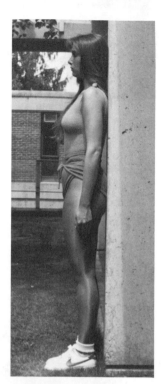

Exercise 7. Wall Press

Objective: To promote good body alignment and posture while strengthening abdominal muscles.

Basic Exercise: Stand erect, with your head and neck in a neutral position, your back against the wall, and your heels 3 inches away from the wall. Suck in your stomach and press your lower back flat against the wall. Hold this position for 6 seconds; relax and return to the starting position. Your lower back should continuously be in contact with the wall and your head and neck should not extend backward.

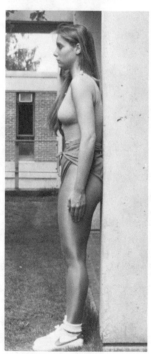

Exercise 8. Posture Check

Objective: To help you stand and walk correctly, and to help you determine if your exercise program is accomplishing its goals.

Basic Exercise: Stand with your back to the wall, pressing your heels, buttocks, shoulders, and head against the wall. You should not be able to feel any space between your lower back and the wall; if you can, your back is too arched and not flat. Move your feet forward, bending your knees so that your back slides a few inches down the wall. Now, again, squeeze your buttocks and tighten your abdominal muscles flattening your lower back against the wall. While holding this position, walk your feet back so you slide up the wall. Now, standing straight, walk away from the wall and around the room. Return to the wall and back up to it to be certain you've kept the proper posture.

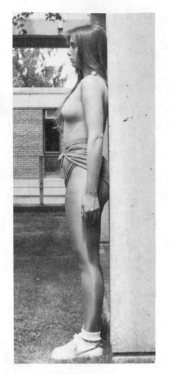

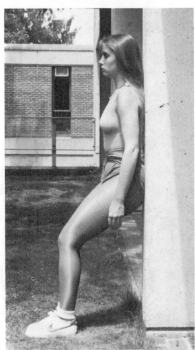

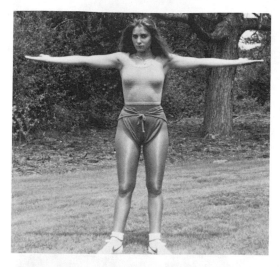

Exercise 9. Arm Circles

Objective: To strengthen the muscles of the shoulder while keeping the joint flexible.

Basic Exercise: Stand erect, with your arms outstretched to the side at shoulder height, palms up. While keeping your head erect, move your hands backward making small circular movements, then reverse and, now with your palms down, carry out the circular movements in a forward circle.

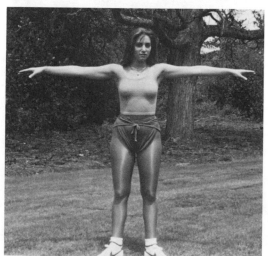

Exercise 10. Half Knee Bend

Objective: To strengthen and stretch your quadriceps (upper front thigh) muscles and improve your balance.

Basic Exercise: Stand erect, with your hands on your hips. Extend your arms forward, palms down, and bend your knees halfway. Keep your heels on the floor, pause, and return to the starting position.

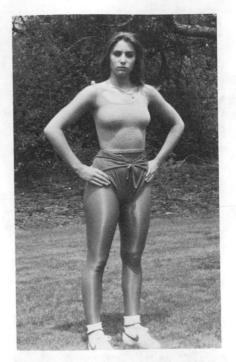

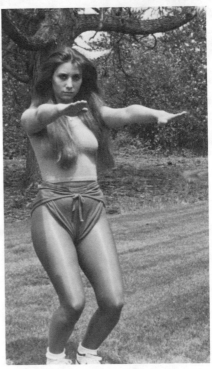

56

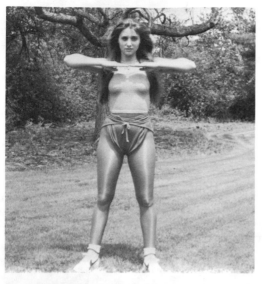

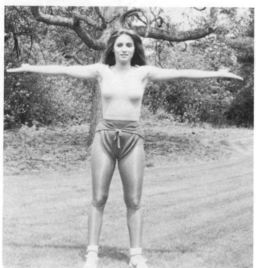

Exercise 11. Wing Stretcher

Objective: To strengthen the muscles of the upper back and shoulders while stretching the chest muscles and promoting good posture.

Basic Exercise: While standing erect, bend your arms in front of your chest, with your elbows at shoulder height and your extended fingertips touching. Count one, two, three; on each count, pull your elbows backward as far as possible while keeping your arms at shoulder height and then returning to the starting position. Then swing your arms (on count four) outward and sideward, shoulder height, palms up, and return to the starting position.

Exercise 12. Wall Push-Up

Objective: To strengthen arm, shoulder, and upper back muscles while stretching the chest and posterior thigh muscles.

Basic Exercise: Stand erect, squarely facing the wall, with your feet about 6 inches apart and your arms extended straight in front, with your palms on the wall lightly bearing weight. Slowly bend your elbows and lower your body toward the wall, turning your head to the side until your cheek almost touches the wall. Then slowly push away from the wall, extending your elbows while returning to the starting position. Then slowly repeat, this time turning your head to the opposite side.

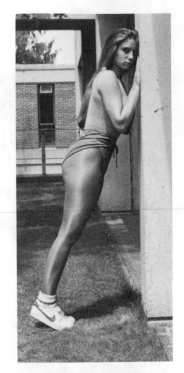

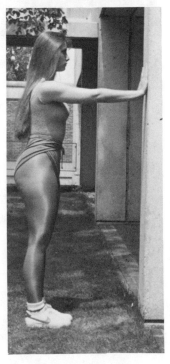

Exercise 13. Single Knee Raise

Objective: To stretch lower back, hip flexor, and hamstring (posterior thigh) muscles.

Basic Exercise: Lie on your back on a padded floor, with your arms above your head and your knees bent. Tighten your buttocks and abdominal muscles as in Exercise 6. Then raise one knee over your chest toward your chin as far as possible, hold for 10 seconds, then return to starting position, and relax a few seconds before repeating with the other. Start with three repetitions of each knee and gradually advance to 10.

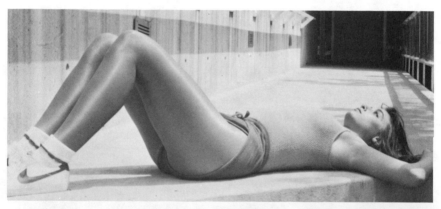

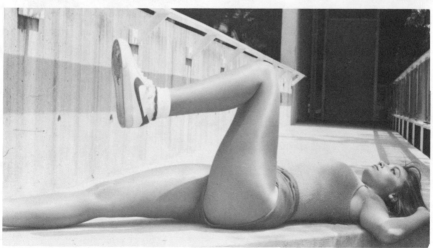

Exercise 14. Single Knee Hug

Objective: Same as single knee raise.

Basic Exercise: The single knee hug is essentially the same exercise as the single knee raise, except that the hands are not placed above the head but rather around the knee that is raised. The arms are used to pull the knee closer to the chest than was possible in Exercise 13. This produces greater stretching of the lower back and hamstrings. The same 10-second hold, number of repetitions, and advanced modification pertain here as with the single knee raise.

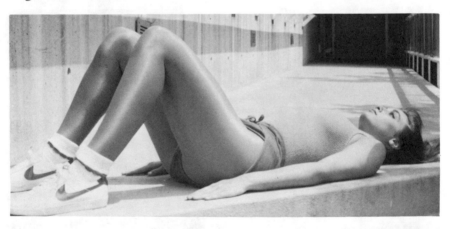

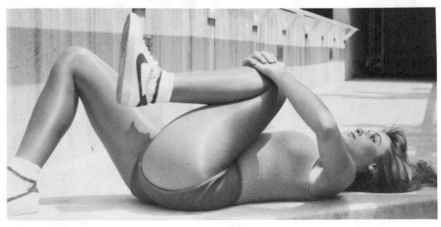

Exercise 15. Double Knee Hug

Objective: To stretch lower back and hamstring muscles and strengthen abdominal and hip-flexing muscles.

Basic Exercise: Lie on your back on a covered floor with knees bent, arms at your side, and pillow under your head, if desired. Tighten your buttocks and abdominal muscles so that your lower back is flat against the floor. Now grasp both knees with your hands and raise them slowly over your chest as far as possible. Hold 10 seconds, return to starting position, relax a few seconds, then repeat. Start with three repetitions and gradually build to 10.

Advanced Modification: After a month or more of the basic exercise, attempt the double knee hug starting with both legs extended straight. Tense your buttocks and abdomen, and then, taking care to keep the back flat, bend both knees, grasp knees with hands and raise over your chest, hold 10 seconds, and return to starting position to relax before repeating. The lower back tends to arch when the knee is lifted and lowered. If you cannot do this with your back against the floor, you are not yet ready for this modification and should resume the basic knees-bent position. This extended leg starting position strengthens both the hip-flexing and abdominal muscles.

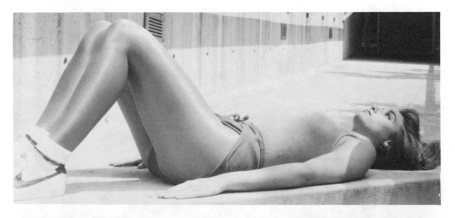

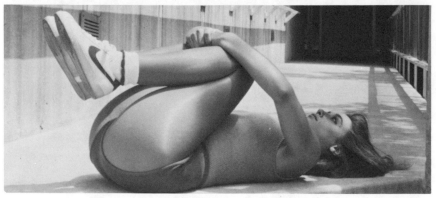

Exercise 16. Single Leg Raise

Objective: To stretch lower back and hamstring muscles and strengthen abdominal and hip-flexing muscles.

Basic Exercise: Lie on your back on a covered floor with one knee bent and one leg straight, arms at your side, and a pillow under your head, if desired. Tighten your buttocks and abdominal muscles, then slowly raise the straight leg, keeping the leg straight and your back flat. Raise the leg as far as comfortably possible, then slowly lower the leg, keeping it straight and your back flat on the floor. Relax a few seconds, and then repeat with the other leg. Start with three repetitions of each leg and gradually increase to 10.

Advanced Modification: After a month or more, attempt the single leg raise starting with both legs extended straight. Tense your buttocks and lower back, and with your back flat and legs out straight, raise one leg up as far as possible. As the leg is raised, your back may not remain flat. Check by using your hand to see if your back lifts from the floor when the leg is lifted and lowered. If it does, resume the basic exercise with one knee bent.

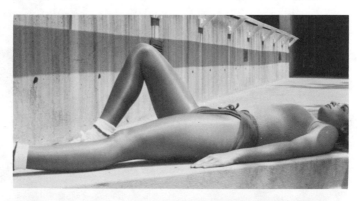

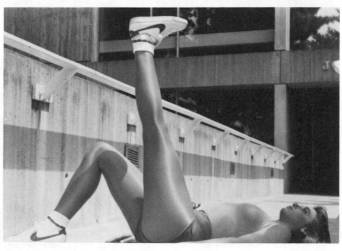

Exercise 17. Single Leg Raise and Knee Hug

Objective: To strengthen lower back and abdominal muscles while increasing flexibility of hip and knee joints.

Basic Exercise: Raise extended left leg about 12 inches off the floor; slowly bend your knee and move it toward your chest as far as possible using your abdominal, hip, and leg muscles. Then place both hands around your knee and pull it slowly toward your chest as far as possible. Slowly extend your leg to the position 12 inches off the floor, then return to the starting position. Repeat 2 to 5 times with each leg. Do the number desired with the left leg, then switch and repeat with the right leg.

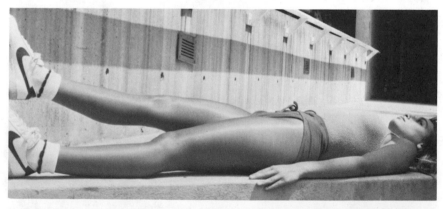

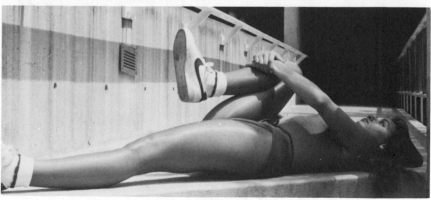

Exercise 18. Straight Arm and Leg Stretch

Objective: To strengthen abdominal muscles while stretching the muscles of the arms.

Basic Exercise: Lie on your back, legs extended, feet together, arms at your side, your buttocks and abdomen tensed so that your back is flat against the floor. Slowly move arms and legs outward along the floor as possible, hold a moment, and slowly return to the starting position. Repetitions as indicated for each level.

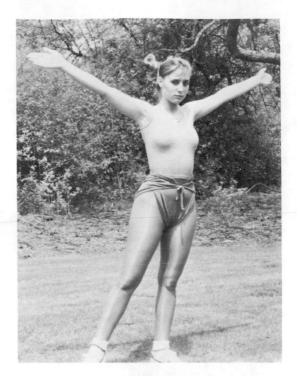

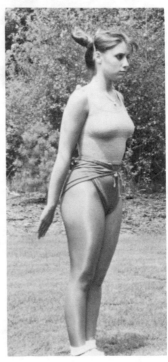

Exercise 19. Heel-Toe Walk

Objective: To improve balance and posture.

Basic Exercise: Stand erect, with abdomen and buttocks tensed, your left foot along a straight line, and your hands held out from your body to aid in balance. Walk 10 steps along the straight line by placing the right foot directly in front of the left, with the right heel touching the left great toe. Then place the left in front of the right, heel-to-toe. When 10 such steps in a straight line have been taken, stop; then return to the starting position by walking backward along the same line, alternately placing one foot behind the other, toe-to-heel.

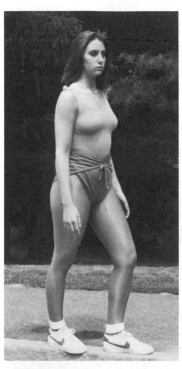

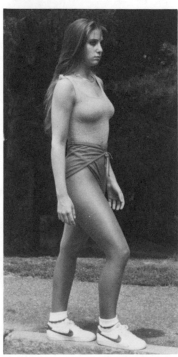

Exercise 20. Heel-Toe Beam Walk

Objective: To improve balance and posture.

Basic Exercise: At Level 2, you will walk 10 steps on a 2-inch-high by 6-inch-wide board placed flat on the floor; at Level 1, use a 2-inch-high by 4-inch-wide board placed flat on the floor. Walk 10 steps along the board by placing the right foot directly in front of the left with the right heel touching the left great toe. Then place the left foot in front of the right, heel-to-toe. When 10 such steps have been taken, stop, then return to the starting position by walking backward along the same board, alternately placing one foot behind the other, toe-to-heel.

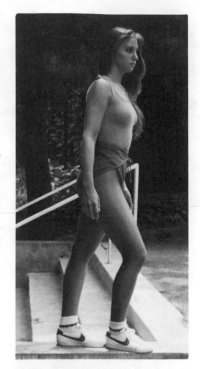

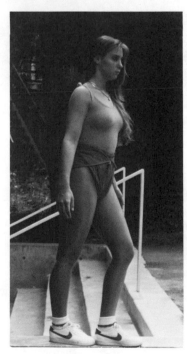

Exercise 21. Hop

Objective: To improve balance, strengthen the extensor muscles of the leg and foot, and increase circulation.

Basic Exercise: Stand erect, lower back flat, with your weight on your right foot, your left leg bent at the knee, and your left foot several inches off the floor. Hold your arms slightly outward from your body to aid in balance. Hop five times on your right foot, and then hop five times on your left foot.

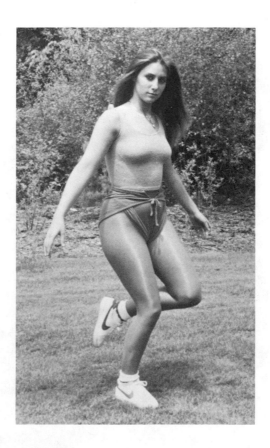

Exercise 22. Knee Push-Up

Objective: To strengthen the muscles of your arms, shoulders, and trunk.

Basic Exercise: Lie on the floor face down, legs together, knees bent, with feet off the floor and your hands palm-down flat on the floor under your shoulders. Slowly push your upper body off the floor, extending your arms fully and keeping your lower back straight so that your body is in a straight line from head to knees. Slowly return to starting position, then repeat.

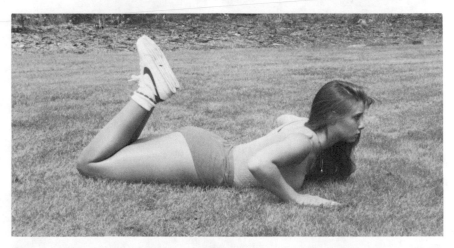

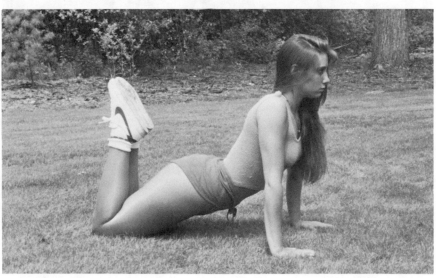

Exercise 23. Side Leg Raise

Objective: To improve the flexibility of the hip joint and strengthen the lateral muscles of the trunk and hip.

Basic Exercise: Lie on the floor on your right side with your head resting on your right arm and both legs extended together. Lift your extended left leg sideways (upward) off the right leg as far as possible. Stop, return to the starting position, and repeat. After the proper number of repetitions are done with the left leg, roll over on your left side and repeat the exercise with your right leg.

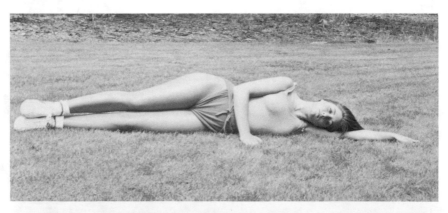

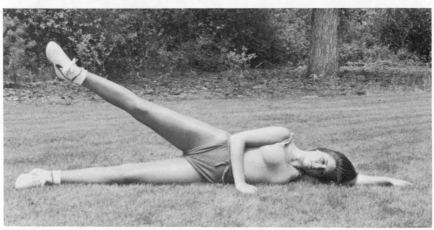

Exercise 24. Partial Sit-Up

Objective: To strengthen lower back and abdominal muscles.

Basic Exercise: Lie on your back on a covered floor with your knees well bent. Tighten your buttocks and your abdominal muscles, with your lower back on the floor, and slowly raise your head, neck, and, finally, shoulders as you extend your arms to your knees. Keep your lower back flat on the floor. Hold this position for 10 seconds, then return to starting position, rest a few seconds, and repeat. Start with three repetitions and work up to at least 10.

Your back will now lift off the floor. Keep your knees bent. In the beginning it may help to place your feet under a heavy chair or some other restraint. Once your abdominal muscles are strong enough, this should not be necessary and should not be done, since this action actually allows your legs to help the abdomen in allowing you to raise. The motion should be a gentle smooth curling and uncurling. Never jerk to achieve greater height or an additional repetition, and never strain or exert yourself beyond reasonable comfort. Again, start with three repetitions and progress to at least 10.

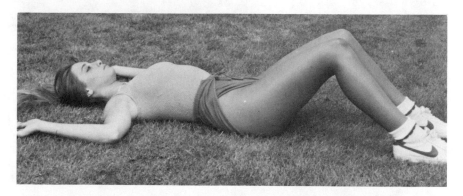

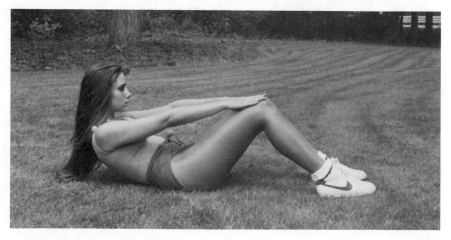

Exercise 25. Advanced Sit-Up

Objective: To maximally strengthen lower back and abdominal muscles.

Basic Exercise: Lie on your back on a covered floor with your knees well bent. Tighten your buttocks and your abdominal muscles. Start with your arms folded over your waist and smoothly lift your head, shoulders, and back up to a position so that your arms are touching your knees. Hold 10 seconds, return to the starting position, relax a few seconds, and then repeat. Again, start with three repetitions and progress to at least 10.

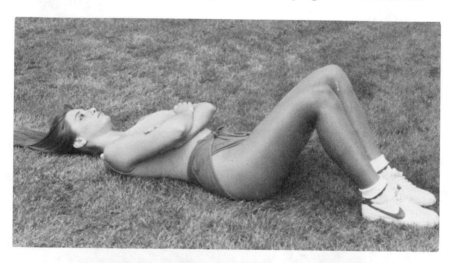

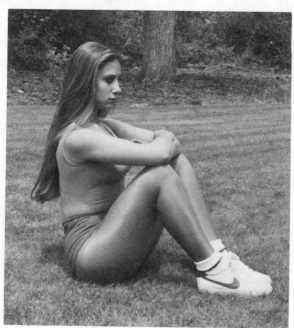

Exercise 26. Advanced Modified Sit-Up

Objective: To maximally strengthen lower back and abdominal muscles.

Basic Exercise: Progress gradually until 10 of the basic advanced sit-ups can be easily and comfortably executed. Then try folding your arms in front of your face instead of your waist. As you curl up to your knees, hold 10 seconds, then return to the starting position, relax a few seconds, and repeat. Start with three repetitions. When this modified version can be accomplished 10 times, you are ready to attempt a sit-up with your hands clasped behind your head. When this version can also be done 10 times, you may attempt the maximal version of a sit-up. This involves lying on your back on a padded inclined surface (i.e., a tilt board with the foot end elevated). Knees should be bent as always, then, with hands clasped behind your neck, slowly and carefully execute the sit-up, hold 10 seconds, slowly uncurl to the starting position, relax, and repeat. This last version is clearly optional. The more inclined the board, the greater strength and effort will be required of your back and abdomen to accomplish the sit-up.

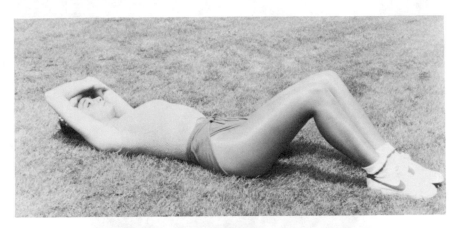

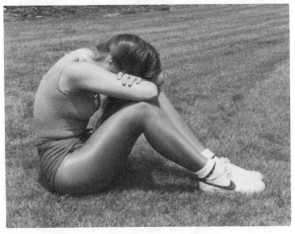

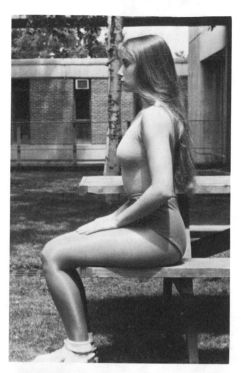

Exercise 27. Sitting Bend

Objective: To strengthen your lower back while stretching your lower back and hamstring muscles.

Basic Exercise: Sit on a hard chair, feet flat on the floor, knees not more than 12 inches apart, arms folded loosely in your lap. Tighten buttocks and abdominal muscles so that your back is flat against the chair. Bend over, letting your head go between your knees, with your hands reaching for the floor. Bend as far as is comfortable, hold for a count of five, then slowly pull your body back to the starting position with your back flat against the chair. Relax a few seconds, then repeat initially three times, gradually increasing to 10 repetitions.

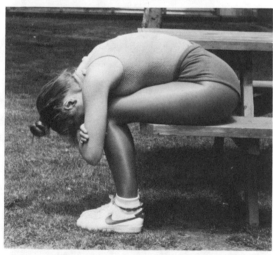

Exercise 28. Diver's Stance

Objective: To improve balance and posture while strengthening extensor muscles of the legs and feet.

Basic Exercise: Stand erect with your buttocks and abdomen tensed, feet slightly apart, and your arms at your sides. Lift up on your toes while extending your arms upward and forward, palms down at shoulder height, parallel to the floor. Hold this position for 10 seconds then return to the starting position and repeat.

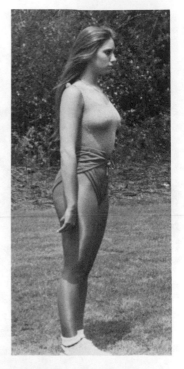

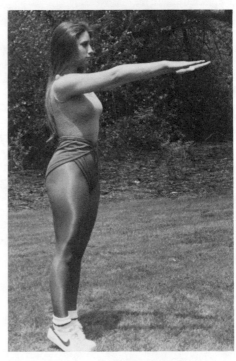

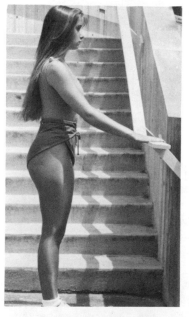

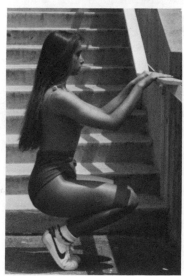

Exercise 29. Deep Knee Bend

Objective: To strengthen the hamstrings and quadriceps muscles.

Caution: Do not begin this exercise until you can do a good Back Flattener. Have someone confirm that you are indeed holding your back flat while executing Exercise 6. Most people should not attempt this exercise until they have been participating in this exercise program for a month. Discontinue this exercise if there is considerable lasting discomfort in your knees or hips, and do not try it if you have a history of knee problems.

Basic Exercise: Stand behind a sofa, desk, or heavy chair, holding onto it for balance. Squeeze and tighten your buttocks and abdomen. Slowly bend your knees and, with a flat back, squat down as far as is reasonably comfortable; stop, then stand up using only your legs and not your arms. Relax for a second or two and then repeat, initially three times, gradually building up to 10 repetitions.

To complete the sequence, repeat Exercise 2, the Alternate Walk-Jog, with the following modifications:
Level 1: Gradually increase to walk 100 steps, then jog 100 steps alternately for 5 minutes.
Level 2: Walk 50 steps, then jog 25 steps alternately for 3 to 6 minutes.
Level 3. Walk 50 steps, then jog 10 steps alternately for 1 to 3 minutes.
Finish with Exercise 1, the walk.

The Daily Regimen

As discussed previously, the essence of physical fitness is a fit cardiovascular system. Having attained Level 1 status, it is now time to liberalize and vary your daily exercise program to make it more stimulating and enjoyable. The rest of this chapter is devoted to showing you how you can do this for yourself. Certain basic concepts, however, should be stressed. For example, your exercise program should include exercises that promote flexibility, coordination, agility, balance, muscular strength, and endurance. Muscles grow soft and atrophy if they are not used. The natural, slow decline of muscular strength and endurance can be retarded only by keeping the muscles toned by means of regular exercise. So, too, the balance and equilibrium mechanisms of the body can be kept fit only through use. The tissue surrounding joints increase in thickness and lose their elasticity with advancing years. This process is greatly retarded by a daily exercise program that moves the joints through the full range of motion. Exercise will keep your joints flexible, your muscles supple and springy, and your heart feeling young.

To be of maximum benefit, your exercise program should be carried out daily. It should have three parts: a *warm-up period,* an *endurance phase,* and a *cooling-off period.* It is analogous to the racehorse warming up, running the race, and returning to the paddock to be cooled off by walking.

The Warm-Up Period

The warm-up period should be at least 5 minutes long and include rhythmic slow stretching movements of the trunk and limb muscles. This increases blood flow and stretches the postural muscles, preparing the body for sustained activity. To ignore the warm-up is to risk muscle pulls or more severe injuries. The list below gives 14 warm-up exercises. You may choose any combination of three for your 5-minute warm-up period. Start with three repetitions and gradually build to 10 or more. Vary the combinations on different days to avoid monotony.

1. Back Flattener (Exercise 6)
2. Single Knee Raise (Exercise 13)
3. Single Knee Hug (Exercise 14)
4. Double Knee Hug (Exercise 15)
5. Single Leg Raise (Exercise 16)

6. Partial Sit-up (Exercise 24)
7. Advanced Sit-up (Exercise 25)
8. Sitting Bend (Exercise 27)
9. Deep Knee Bend (Exercise 29)
10. Posture Check (Exercise 8)
11. Bend and Stretch (Exercise 3)
12. Wall Push-up (Exercise 12)
13. Hop 3 minutes (Exercise 21)
14. Diver's Stance (Exercise 28)

The Endurance Phase

The endurance phase should last at least 15 to 30 minutes. During this period your cardiovascular system is stressed to increase aerobic capacity. What are the best cardiovascular exercises for you? It has been said that the best exercise is the one you most enjoy because it is the one you will most likely continue to do. Certain characteristics are desirable and, thus, make some exercises more beneficial than others.

First, from a cardiovascular standpoint, the primary objective is sustained vigorous exercise pursued for a length of time sufficient to burn more than 400 calories. *Sustained* means that the exercise must be done continuously without stopping. If you plan to exercise for 30 or more minutes, do not stop once during that period of time. Already you can guess that a sport such as football, with a huddle between every play, would rank low as a fitness exercise pursuit. The activity should increase your heart rate to approximately 74 to 80% of its maximal potential in order for you to experience cardiovascular improvement. For most of us, this translates into a pulse rate of about 120 to 150 beats per minute to achieve this increased endurance fitness. Practically speaking, this also translates into a 75 to 80% maximal oxygen consumption. To exceed 80% of maximal cardiac output as measured by pulse rate may lead to inadequate oxygenation; that is, you cannot consume oxygen fast enough, so your body shifts to anaerobic or nonoxygen metabolism, which may cause tissue damage. In reality, most exercise is achieved at a lower pulse rate.

Another feature of endurance involves the ability to increase the workload as your level of fitness increases. With increased fitness, the same activity that initially caused a pulse rate of 140 may now produce an increase to only 100. Thus, the activity must be made progressively more difficult. This can be accomplished in one of two ways. You can slowly increase the overall rate at which you carry out the exercise. The progress should be accomplished in many small steps. Or you can introduce intervals of a faster pace alternating with a slower pace. The faster pace should be sufficiently vigorous so that you incur an oxygen debt; then switch to a slower pace in order to replenish your oxygen supply. Competitive athletes use interval training extensively, but you will probably prefer to increase your pace slowly at a comfortable rate as your fitness progresses.

Table 4-3
Energy Expenditures for Moderate Activities

Recreational Activities
(400–600 calories burned/hour)

Badminton*	Curling*	Skating*	Touch football
Baseball	Dancing*	Skindiving	Volleyball*
Bicycling	Deck tennis*	Softball	Walking
(~10mph)*	Fencing	Squash	(~5mph on level)*
Canoeing*	Paddle tennis	Table tennis*	Water skiing†
Cricket	Rowing*	Tennis*†	

Household Activities
(4–6 calories per minute for a 150-pound person.
To be used as an endurance workout, these activities must be pursued
very vigorously in a nonstop manner for 60–75 minutes.)

Mowing the lawn with a hand mower	Walking up small hills
Hoeing	Walking in water
Spading the garden	Walking in loose sand on a level
Raking leaves	Pushing a loaded wheelbarrow
Pulling weeds	Carrying 30–50 pounds on a level
Playing a musical instrument	Painting requiring a ladder
energetically	Cutting hedges with hand clipper
Sawing wood by hand	Sanding wood, metal, etc.
Splitting logs by hand	Light-moderate activities done
Vigorously mopping or scrubbing floors	vigorously

*Recommended for persons over 50 by the International Committee on the Standardization of Physical Fitness.
†Should be approached cautiously by those with back problems.
**From *Diabetes and Exercise* by Robert C. Cantu, M.D., F.A.C.S. Copyright © 1982 by Robert C. Cantu. Reprinted by permission of the publisher, E. P. Dutton, Inc.

Tables 4-2, 4-3 and 4-4 classify sports as heavy, moderate, or light-moderate, according to their exercise value and the energy output they require. A number of household projects are also graded and can be substituted in the exercise program as endurance activities. In the heavy exercise group, these include chopping wood, shoveling snow, and digging holes; in the moderate group, scrubbing floors and performing heavy gardening chores like mowing the lawn or pulling weeds; in the light-moderate group, sweeping floors, ironing, washing clothes, making beds, and doing light work in the garden.

A few comments on the relative merits of various activities seem appropriate to this discussion. In my opinion, the finest three activities for total

Table 4-4
Energy Expenditures For Light-Moderate Activities

Recreational Activities
(200–400 calories burned/hour)

Archery*	Croquet*	Horseback riding*	Shuffleboardq*
Baseball	Fishing*	Horseshoes*†	Walking
Bowling*†	Golf*	Sailing*	(~5mph on level)*

Household Activities
(1–3 calories per minute for a 150-pound person.
To be used as an endurance workout, these activities must be pursued
very vigorously in a nonstop manner for 1½–2 hours.)

Making the bed	Making minor repairs on the car
Cleaning the tub	Building with wood
Ironing clothes	Painting
Putting away groceries	Shampooing rugs with an electric
Vacuuming the floor or pool	cleaner
Dusting	Walking on a level or downhill
Washing clothes by hand	surface
Washing floors, walls, or windows	Raking leaves
Light gardening	Paperhanging
Mowing the lawn with a power	Bricklaying
mower	Cleaning windows
Pruning bushes	Light carpentry
Cutting hedges with an electric cutter	Janitorial work
Washing or waxing the car by hand	Sewing, knitting
	Playing a musical instrument

*Recommended for persons over 50 by the International Committee on the Standardization of Physical Fitness.
†Should be approached cautiously by those with back problems.
**From *Diabetes and Exercise* by Robert C. Cantu, M.D., F.A.C.S. Copyright © 1982 by Robert C. Cantu, Reprinted by permission of the publisher, E. P. Dutton, Inc.

body conditioning are swimming, cross-country skiing, and roller skiing. Unlike jogging, which does little to strengthen or increase upper-body joint flexibility, each of these three combines a vigorous cardiovascular endurance workout with strengthening and increased flexibility of all the joints. On the negative side, swimming is boring for many, cross-country skiing requires snow, and roller skiing does subject one to the risks of falling. The second tier of ideal sports for conditioning (the heavy exercise gorup) includes jogging, cycling, rope skipping, and rowing. Jogging and rope skipping are the least expensive and most expedient. Cycling and rowing may each involve a large initial outlay of money, and cycling, if practiced on city streets, can be dangerous.

The great advantage of this fitness program is that you can tailor it to your own likes and dislikes. Practically any vigorous physical activity can be used in the endurance phase, provided it is performed for a long enough period of time and with sufficient intensity. For example, a weekend ski trip or a vigorous tennis match can count for one of the required workouts. Or you can substitute hard physical labor, like shoveling snow or sawing wood, for one of the endurance periods. If you enjoy sports, then on any given day you can substitute 30 minutes of maximal exercise sports (e.g., running, stationary running, cycling, cross-country skiing, or swimming), 60 mintues of moderate sports activity (e.g., tennis, skiing), or 90 minutes of minimal exericse sports (e.g., golf, gardening, canoeing, bowling, fishing, archery, horseshoes, ping-pong, shuffleboard, or social dancing). The time periods, of course, can be as long as you want.

Whichever exercise you select from the tables, the primary emphasis should be on *safe* and *enjoyable* participation. Since few will adhere to an exercise commitment that is not pleasurable, it is best to do whatever you most enjoy. On those days when the weather is poor outside or when you cannot exercise in daylight, you may substitute if necessary the indoor activities of jogging in place, walking stairs, rope skipping, stationary bicycle riding, etc.

The Cooling-Off Period

The cooling-off period is the reverse of the warm-up period by helping your body return to normal. It should be at least 5 minutes long and should consist of rhythmic slow stretching movements of the trunk and limb muscles. Neglecting the cooling-off period can result in light-headedness, dizziness, nausea and fainting. Also, the cooling-off period drains your muscles of the lactic acid which has accumulated during the endurance phase. This prepares the body for strenuous exercise the next day and eases any muscle soreness which might occur. See the warm-up list of exercises on pages 76–77. You may choose any combination of three for your 5 minute cooling-off period. Start with three repititions and gradually build to 10 or more. Change the combination to avoid monotony.

Section II

Special Considerations

Chapter 5

Sports Injuries in Young Athletes

Young athletes are not merely small adults. Because they possess immature bones and ligaments that can easily be overstressed, they incur different types of acute sports injuries. The problems they present are unique.

The normal growth and development of children has enormous variation in stages of development at any one time. The average weight of an 11-year-old boy is 78 pounds, but a child's weight may vary from 50 to 108 pounds and still be within the "normal" range. The maturation of the nervous system, which results in coordination of large muscle groups, may also vary vastly for a given age. And the maturity factor must be considered. A 14-year-old boy may exhibit very little pubertal change or he may be fully developed. Since muscle power, coordination, and oxygen consumption develop rapidly with the hormonal changes of puberty, especially in boys, the prepubertal athlete is at a significant disadvantage when competing with the postpubertal athlete, even if both are the same size. All of the above factors have obvious implications in contact or collision sports. Coaches, trainers, and team physicians must keep this in mind when selecting and matching teams for competition in contact sports. Fortunately for the pre–high school athlete, collision injuries are usually minor because they occur at a slow speed. However, this is no longer the case by high school age, and as a result both the number and severity of collision injuries increase, with the lighter, smaller, less physically mature athlete being the major recipient.

Athletes as a group are impatient about restrictions that an injury may impose. But young athletes, lacking judgment and experience, are the least

83

likely to follow recommended limitations of activity, even when they are essential for the proper diagnosis and healing of injuries. Therefore, it is prudent to exercise an extremely close follow-up regimen for the injured young athlete and to anticipate impatient behavior.

Open bone growth centers and flexible ligamentous structures result in musculoskeletal injuries unique to the young athlete that require prompt orthopedic evaluation and treatment.

Epiphyseal Injury

Bones lengthen primarily by growth in the cartilage of the growth center (epiphyseal plate). Once growth has occurred in the cartilage, the cartilage degenerates and is replaced by new bone. This new bone is much weaker than mature bone. Thus, the growing bone of the young athlete has an inherent area of weakness due to the very processes of growth. The growth centers have less resistance to sheer, compressive, and tensile forces than do adjacent bone. While most growth center fractures heal without a problem, all should be handled by an orthopedic surgeon, because injury may result in permanent growth arrest with deformity. Ages 12 to 13 are the prime ages for this type of injury. The growth center of the radius at the wrist is the most commonly injured bone. Such injuries may be passed off as sprains. The key to proper recognition is a high index of suspicion and the persistence of pain and tenderness for more than 48 hours.

Growth center injuries can also occur in young athletes because their ligaments are stronger than the new bone of the growth center. Thus, in joints where a ligament attaches to the growth center per se, injuries that would normally result in a ligamentous injury in the adult often result in growth center fractures in young athletes. The knee, ankle, and elbow are especially prone to this injury, which requires orthopedic evaluation.

Apophyseal Injury

The apophyseal centers are eminences, tubercles, or other protruberances on bones where major muscle tendons insert. They have separate areas of growth that allow them to enlarge as the tendons increase in size. The growth occurs much the same way as in the epiphyseal plate. Thus, they represent another area of weakness. The apophyses can become partially or completely separated from the bone when large muscle forces are suddenly applied. In the adult hamstring muscle, ruptures occur with hyperflexion (overbending) of the hip combined with an extended knee. In the skeletally immature young athlete, the ischial apophysis may be torn away instead. Other apophyses that may incur a similar injury are in the pelvis, upper leg, iliac crest (a part of the pelvis), and hip. Apophyseal injury, if unrecognized and thus untreated, may result in significant physical impairment.

84

Ligament and Tendon Injuries

Because the ligaments and tendons of the young athlete are more flexible than those of the adult, strains are less common, but they do occur. Micro-tears of a tendon with resulting hemorrhage may be seen in the young athlete involving the patellar tendon of the knee where it attaches to either the inferior pole of the patella (kneecap) (Sinding-Larson syndrome) or to the tibial (large leg bone) tubercle (Osgood-Schlatter's Disease), or where the Achilles heel tendon attaches to the apophysis of the calcaneus (ankle) (Seiver's Disease). Most of these syndromes respond to varying periods of rest.

Young athletes may also possess unrecognized congenital conditions that place them at increased risk for athletic injury. Many of these defects weaken the bone (e.g., unicameral bone cyst, fibrous dysplasia, and non-ossifying fibromas). Therefore, whenever a young athlete incurs a fracture with minimal trauma, such a lesion should be suspected.

Young athletes usually lack the motivation to work diligently to thoroughly condition their bodies for endurance, strength, and acclimatization to heat. Thus, the coach, trainer, or team physician has to motivate the young athlete to properly condition him- or herself not only to achieve maximal performance, but also to minimize risk of injury.

Indifference about the fitting, adjustment, and care of their protective equipment is common in our youth. Protective equipment, especially in contact and collision sports, is designed to prevent injury. It will not only fail to function if improperly fitted, but it may directly cause injury. Since it is vital to the health and success of young athletes, coaches, trainers, and team physicians must educate them in the proper fitting, maintenance, and usage of equipment. Full equipment must always be employed in contact and collision sports, whether it be practice or a game. Any equipment used in practice should be mandatory for a game. If a knee pad or extra hip padding is used in a game, it must be used in practice and vice versa. Coaches, trainers, and team physicians must constantly check that full protective equipment and any necessary special equipment is always used during games and practice alike. Failure to do so will eventually lead to needless injury.

Young athletes frequently lack the supervision and advice of a qualified athletic trainer. These duties are usually assumed by a coach or parent or by a physician who frequently may be available only by phone. Many worrisome problems would be alleviated if certified athletic trainers were universally available to oversee the health of our young athletes.

Risk Factors

The primary factor in the production of injuries in young athletes is the inherent violence of the sport itself. Thus, the injury rate in football and wrestling is far greater than that in tennis or swimming. The American Academy of Pediatrics found injuries occurring in young athletes most often in football, wrestling, gymnastics, basketball, ice hockey, and lacrosse. But before we denounce contact or collision sports for young athletes, we should note that surveys show the incidence of injuries in unsupervised play activities such as bicycling, skateboarding, and skating to be much higher than in supervised football or soccer. Even football, the sport with the highest rate of injury, the most serious injuries (fractures, injuries to the knee, etc.), and the most hospitalizations is far safer per hour of exposure than riding in a car.

A second factor in injury risk is the age, size, and maturity of the young athlete. As size and age increase, speed increases, and thus the violence of collision and contact is enhanced. Therefore, the high school athlete is at greatest risk of injury, the junior high athlete next, and the grade school athlete least. While more boys are injured than girls, this is a result of the sports selected, and sex is not a factor in the injury rate for sports with equal participation. Furthermore, in the prepubertal age group, sex is not a factor in determining injury predisposition or in performance.

The risk of injury to specific body parts is highest for the head, fingers, knees, and ankles. The lower back is especially prone to injury in gymnastics. The risk of permanent injury is low, about 1% of all injuries, with the knee being the most vulnerable area of the body.

Injury Prevention

The avoidance of injury in young athletes starts with a comprehensive sports health examination. The medical history should elucidate potential problems that might rule out the sport in question, and the athlete's fitness and maturation level should be assessed. All accidents, injuries, illnesses, or operations that may conceivably affect an athlete's performance in a given sport must be examined. Treatable conditions should be discovered and a plan of treatment implemented. While a complete physical examination for each sport is certainly unnecessary, the sports health history should be mandatory for each sport. Table 5-1 is an example of a health history form. Barring injury or illness, the athlete's physical examination may be done annually by a primary care physician or pediatrician and supplemented with periodic health history appraisals for each sport. Any injury or illness would, of course, require medical clearance with respect to that problem before resumption of competition.

A second major factor in injury prevention is education—the proper way to play the sport, how to wear the equipment, and so on. A recent study reported nearly a third of all sports injuries in the young are avoidable. Young athletes must be educated by coaches, trainers, and physicians in the proper fitting, use, and maintenance of their equipment. They must realize that equipment that is used to prevent injury, when improperly fitted or used, can cause injury. Since most injuries occur in practice, full use of equipment is mandatory for practice. Any equipment worn in a game setting should be worn in practice.

The most glaring misuse of equipment is the use of the football helmet to spear or butt-block in football. Now declared illegal when detected, these practices were responsible for a rash of cervical spine fracture dislocations and quadriplegias, especially in high school football in the 1970s.

While recognizing the impossibility of all youth sports activities being conducted under optimal conditions, the Committee on Pediatric Aspects of Physical Fitness, Recreation, and Sports suggested that the following be implemented whenever possible:

1. Medical care should always be readily available. If a physician or athletic trainer cannot be on-site, he or she should be readily available.

2. Prior to the first practice session, preparation for the care of injuries should be planned and implemented. Medical and other emergency materials must be promptly available.

3. The physician and/or athletic trainer must have sole authority to make decisions regarding management of medical care and return to play after injury.

4. Management of injuries must never be based on expediency, but rather on sound medical judgment and practice. No matter how severe the pressure to make concessions, none must ever be made.

5. While tradition normally excludes the physician from the playing field until summoned, this should not apply to the young athlete. If potentially permanent injuries are to be avoided, immediate care and prompt diagnosis are essential. Before the athlete is transported from the playing field, the physician should speak with the injured athlete and, if necessary, other players and officials to learn how the injury was incurred.

Table 5-1*
Health History Assessment Suggested
For Sports Physical Examination

(To be completed by parent or student before student participation in each competitive sport.)

You must have had a:
I. Complete physical exam within the last two years
   date of exam _____
   name of physician _____
   positive findings   none _____ yes _____
   if *yes,* list _____

II. Do you have now, or have you had	No	Yes
1) loss of eye, lung, kidney, ovary, or testis	____	____
2) loss of vision or hearing	____	____
3) a seizure, convulsion, or epileptic attack	____	____

   4) suggested you have a brain wave test
(EEG, electroencephalogram)   ——   ——
   5) loss of consciousness
     if *yes,* check which one   ——   ——
     A. knocked out   ——   ——
     B. passed out, blacked out, fainted   ——   ——
       Were you hospitalized?   ——   ——
   6) a concussion
     if *yes*   ——   ——
     A. how many times?   ——
     B. how long before complete recovery?   ——
     C. how many games missed after concussion?   ——
   7) a skull fracture   ——   ——
   8) a spine fracture (neck or back)   ——   ——
   9) an x-ray of neck or spine   ——   ——
 10) an injury producing weakness or numbness
of either your arms or legs   ——   ——
 11) a "pinched nerve"   ——   ——
 12) suffered from heat exhaustion   ——   ——
 13) diabetes, congenital heart disease, rheumatic
heart disease, or other serious illness
in the past year   ——   ——
 14) are you currently taking any medicines
or drugs?   ——   ——
     if *yes*
     A. What medication and dose _____
     B. Why? _____

III. Since last exam have you had any injury to:
   head   none   ——   yes   ——
   eyes   ——   ——
   neck   ——   ——
   chest   ——   ——
   back   ——   ——
   abdomen   ——   ——
   arms, legs   ——   ——
   kidneys   ——   ——
   genitals   ——   ——

     If yes, please have a physician complete this section of the form in
regard to this injury.

Nature of injury _____
Any disability   none   ——   yes   ——
If so, what _____
Comment or recommendation
                none   ——   yes   ——

If so, what _____

Date of exam _____

Signature of M.D. _____

IV. Physical Fitness Test:

You must be able to successfully complete the following test before you can engage in any competitive sport.

	Boy	Girl
1) mile	(walk, run) in 8 min.	mile (walk, run) in 10 min.
2) sit-ups		
age 10–12	35	age 10 and over—20
age 13–14	55	
age 15 and over	60	
3) 50-yd. dash		
age 10–12	8.5 sec.	age 10 and over—9.0 sec.
age 13–15	7.6 sec.	
age 15 and over	7.0 sec.	

I agree to the above conditions in order to engage in _____

Signature of Student _____

Upon completion of the above, I give permission for _____
to compete in _____

Signature of Parent _____

Date _____

*Based on NAJPER Youth Fitness Test Manual and Aerobic by Dr. Cooper

*Reproduced with permission from *Sports Injuries, The Unthwarted Epidemic,* edited by Paul F. Vinger and Earl F. Hoerner. © 1981 Wright-PSG Publishing Co., Inc.

Special Physical Considerations

The young student-athlete obviously must be viewed in a different light than the professional whose livelihood depends on his or her performance. Certain conditions, therefore, must be considered to alter or exclude participation in a given sport. For instance, the absence of a paired internal organ (e.g., kidney, testis) or one eye should eliminate participation in collision or contact sports (boxing, football, ice hockey, lacrosse, rugby). This would not prevent participation in any number of other non–contact-collision sports (e.g., baseball, golf, tennis, running, swimming, etc.). For the young athlete with one eye, in addition to contact-collision sports, those sports with a high likelihood of face injury (such as racquet sports) are to be avoided.

The subject of a concussion is discussed in chapter 11. It suffices to say here that two grade II concussions or one grade III concussion should eliminate the return to competition during that season. The young athlete must be asymptomatic at maximal exertion before returning to competition after a concussion.

Following a febrile illness (e.g., virus, otitis media, bronchitis, sinusitis), it is recommended that the young athlete be without fever for 48 hours before resuming strenuous athletic activity. With mononucleosis, the recovery will be much longer. No contact is to be allowed until the spleen has returned to normal size with this condition.

Disability under control is not a contraindication for any sports. The same is true for the young person with idiopathic seizure disorder who is under good control and who has had no seizures for over a year (on medication). Most people with asthma can participate in all sports, unless their asthma is exercise induced. Endurance sports are contraindicated in athletes whose asthma is exercise induced. By the time a child is 10, almost all congenital heart conditions that would preclude sports participation have been diagnosed. This leaves a large number of young athletes with heart murmurs without heart disease. It has been estimated that 30 to 50% of all children will at one time or another have a heart murmur (Murray). Most of these innocent heart murmurs are of short duration, always systolic, and may be present or absent from time to time in the same child. While the pediatric cardiologist has the final say, there is no reason to restrict the athletic activity of a child with an innocent heart murmur.

Psychological Considerations for the Young Athlete

The psychological needs of the young athlete are the same as for older athletes, only more so. Young athletes require positive input and approval at frequent intervals; this is even more true for competitive athletes. Yet, what we find all too often in organized youth sports programs is adults acting like children when children do not play like adults. Put a whistle, a baseball cap, and jersey with the words "coach" on some adults, and they forget that young athletes require frequent praise and need to be treated with respect. Instead, adults sometimes feel—wrongly—that because these young people are "athletes" they need discipline, criticism, and intimidation. A young player who is criticized in public by his coach is learning nothing of positive value. We are aware of the primary negative reasons why young athletes quit a sport. They include:

1. NOT GETTING TO PLAY

While it may seem harsh to "cut" a young athlete from a team, it is far more cruel to allow him to expend exhausting amounts of time and energy in practice and not participate in games. Surveys have shown that young athletes value playing more than winning. More than 90% of the young athletes questioned responded they would rather play on a losing team than ride the bench of a winning team.

2. MISMATCHING

As we discussed before, the physical maturation of the young athlete varies widely, especially in the 10- to 16-year age range. Two boys the same age may vary up to 60 months in skeletal age. When young athletes are significantly mismatched, the smaller, skeletally immature youth finds no enjoyment in constantly being defeated and physically abused by a much larger opponent. And finding no enjoyment and his safety at risk, it is no wonder the severely mismatched youth leaves the sport.

3. NEGATIVE REINFORCEMENT

While negative reinforcement and criticism may transiently motivate young athletes to try harder, over a period of time constant criticism turns them off. As is true for adults, the young athlete must learn new techniques and skills, and this process will occur at varying rates. No one wishes to be made to feel inadequate during this period, and everyone wants to have progress acknowledged. The coach, rather than pointing out what a young athlete is doing wrong, should instruct him or her in the proper way to execute the activity.

4. OVERORGANIZATION

Practices can become so regimented that the young athlete is deprived of the most powerful incentive for sport, *fun*. When it ceases to be fun, young people will likely turn their attention elsewhere.

5. PSYCHOLOGICAL STRESS

High levels of stress can also eliminate fun from sports for the young athlete. This is especially true when young athletes perceive that more is being demanded of them—whether by parents, coaches, peers, or themselves—than is realistically attainable.

6. FAILURE

Constantly losing, especially when they are reminded of failures by coaches, parents, or peers, also eradicates fun from sports for the young athlete. We all wish to feel successful and worthy. Repeated failure creates anxiety, lessens motivation, and reduces performance and feelings of self-esteem. It is no wonder the young athlete who is made to feel or perceives himself or herself as a failure in a given sport will quit the activity.

While the psychological needs of the young athlete are not unique, each youngster is unique as a person. He or she varies in physical and psychological maturity, response to criticism, perceptions as to what is stressful, and goals derived from sports. These differences play an important role in determining the readiness for participation, degree of involvement, and enjoyment received from sports. Because of these variables, no specific one best age can be given for all young athletes to begin sports competition, but some guidelines are available. For young people who mature at a normal rate: 6 years noncontact (e.g., swimming, tennis, track, and field); 8 years contact (basketball, soccer, wrestling); 10 years collision (ice hockey, lacrosse, football). Guidelines aside, perhaps the best indication of when a child is ready to compete is when he or she, without any adult influence, spontaneously expresses a desire to participate in a given sport. Furthermore, it is recommended that the initial intensity of competition be low and increase as skill and interest increase. If matched for size and maturity, most young athletes will find sports to be exhilarating, challenging, safe, and enjoyable.

Chapter 6

Senior Athletes

The November 1977 cover of *Runner's World* shows a picture of John A. Kelley, smiling, with arms outstretched, crossing the finish line of the Falmouth 7.2-mile road race. The caption reads, "Will you look this alive on your 70th birthday?" Since the life span of the average American male is about 67 years, you may question whether you will even be alive at 70. Yet, the happiness in John's face and his lean muscular body testify to the positive effects of vigorous physical activity. John has now run competitive races for over half a century. His first Boston Marathon was in 1928, and he has run more Boston Maratthons (51) than any other person. He won the event twice, in 1935 and in 1945, and holds seven age-group records. Today, 5 years later at age 75, he continues to run about an hour a day on the roads or beach near his Cape Cod home. He still races more than 15 times a year and says, "I'm still enjoying my training, very, very much."

But, you may say, "I am over 60 and have not vigorously exercised since my school years. I wish I had lived the life of John A. Kelley, but what can I possibly do now?" Well, today is the first day of the rest of your life! You will be a long time dead, but while you are alive you are never too old to attain physical fitness! Just take a note of a 70-year-old patient who was medically evaluated just prior to his attempt to break the world age record for the mile run. This man had attended school through the 11th grade, but had never participated on any school teams or been involved with organized running. He worked for 40 years as a machinist. At the age of 60, he joined a YMCA exercise class and began with calisthenics and 1 mile of running each week. Gradually he increased his running and actually competed in the Boston Marathon for five consecutive years. Prior to his mile run, this elderly gentleman underwent exercise stress testing with oxygen uptake analysis, the objective testing of cardiovascular fitness. The oxygen consumption recorded was the highest ever achieved in his age group. On June 9, 1973, he ran in an AAU sanctioned 1-mile race. His time of

6 minutes, 13 seconds (6:13) easily broke the prior age record of 6:55 set in 1969. The former record-holder, now 76 years young, finally had his record broken by an individual who had never seriously exercised until he was 60 years young!

Why cite these two over-65 runners? Am I trying to turn all of you into serious runners? No, I am merely pointing out that if God gave you an unusually endowed body, you can resurrect it at almost any age short of the grave. Even if you are not so endowed—and 95% of the population of this country is not—you can still look forward to physical fitness and participation in athletics.

The retirement years should be happy ones, yet only those who are healthy, alert, and active can appreciate them fully. Yet, even if you enter your 60s with five prior decades of inadequate physical activity, you can still regain and maintain an active, lively way of life. Just as energy begets energy, similarly the only way to increase your own level of energy is to increase your activity. To *keep* lively you must *be* lively!

This chapter presents a plan to increase your current level of physical fitness. How fit you become will depend on the amount of movement you are willing and able to undertake. Research has shown us that cardiovascular fitness can be attained at any age and that women advance as rapidly as men.

You may ask, "Why exercise in my final years?" The answer is found in the contention of most medical authorities that regardless of age, exercise makes a person look, feel, and work better. Exercise stimulates the various bodily functions, especially the digestive process. It improves posture and, through appropriate low-back exercises, it can eliminate low pain and disability. Physical activity also reduces most coronary risk factors including hypercholesterolemia, hypertension, and obesity. In addition, the well-conditioned person usually develops a positive self-image. Feeling more confidence in your body encourages you to thrust yourself into new and stimulating experiences. As a physically fit elderly person, you can look forward to a high degree of independence. Perhaps it is this quality of independence that is to be most prized in later years. The financial and psychological advantages are obvious in being able to plan and do things without leaning on relatives, friends, or paid help. To drive your own car, to succeed with do-it-yourself projects rather than paying someone else for the service, to come and go as you please, to be an asset rather than a liability in emergencies—these are forms of personal freedom well worth striving for.

The basis of physical fitness in later years, as at any age, is a fit cardiovascular system. In addition, senior athletes have other special concerns. As we advance in age, our muscles, tendons, and ligaments, if not used daily, tend to become tighter and less flexible, so it is easier to sustain strains and sprains. It is especially important that our exercise program specifically promote flexibility, coordination, agility, balance, muscular strength, and endurance. Muscles, if not used, grow soft and atrophy. The natural, slow decline of muscular strength and endurance can be retarded only by keeping our muscles toned through regular exercise. So too, the balance and equilibrium mechanisms of the body can be kept fit only through use, and accelerated degeneration occurs with disuse. The tissue surrounding our joints increases in thickness and loses its elasticity with advancing years. This process is greatly retarded (as is arthritis) by a daily exercise program that moves the joints through the full range of motion. Contrary to prevailing notions, our senior citizens should be encouraged to bend, move, and stretch, because exercise will keep their joints flexible, their muscles supple and springy, and their hearts feeling young.

To be of maximum benefit, an exercise program for seniors must be carried out daily or nearly so. It should begin with an extended warm-up period that includes some easy stretching, pulling, and rotating movements. The warm-up should be longer (15 to 20 minutes) and more gentle than for younger athletes. This can be safely followed by a period of more vigorous physical activity, which should be broken up by times of less strenuous exercise. Great care should be taken that this endurance period not be too excessive too frequently. Overuse injuries are more easily sustained in this age group. Thus, a hard workout should not be attempted more than once or twice a week. Many also find it easier to concentrate on the lower body one day, as with running or bicycling, and the upper body the next, as with rowing. As is true at any age, the only way to improve your physical strength and conditioning is to systematically and slowly increase the physical work load. Once you can comfortably carry out a given physical exercise, say five times, the next step is to do it six times, and so on. This same exercise principle applies to the conditioning of the cardiovascular-pulmonary system. To increase the efficiency of the heart and lungs, it is essential to perform continuous rhythmic exercises long enough to stress the cardiovascular-pulmonary system. Thus, brisk walking, jogging, bicycling, or cross-country skiing, for example, should be maintained until the body begins to perspire and the pulse rate rises above 130 beats a minute for several minutes. Within 10 minutes after exertion, your pulse rate should return to normal and you should not feel fatigued. If this does not occur, you are advancing too fast. Many of our senior athletes may already have been exercising for many years, and their goals may well be just to maintain their already accrued levels of fitness.

Determining Your Level of Fitness

What is a sensible exercise program for you? Obviously, this depends on your present health and level of cardiovascular fitness. It is recommended that you begin with a general physical examination and stress electro-cardiogram. Ideally, your physician should be knowledgeable about aerobic exercising and can assist you in arriving at a starting point. However, if you do not have this luxury, you can determine your own level of fitness by several easy tests as discussed in Chapter 4.

To be of maximum value, your exercises should be done daily. A half hour should be sufficient time. Start easily and slowly, increasing the tempo and number of repetitions. If you feel a little stiff, do not let this deter you. However, if you experience frank pain that does not disappear in 48 hours, delete that exercise until it can be resumed without pain or until medical clearance is given. The exercises in Levels 1, 2, and 3, as discussed in Chapter 4, should be carried out in the sequence given, as both a warm-up and cooling-off period are built into each series. The cooling-off period has recently received much attention in the Olympic games. It is the cooling-off phase that allows your muscles to be drained of lactic acids, the products of anaerobic metabolism. This is the best way to prepare the body for strenuous activity the next day. If possible, you should keep a log or record of the exercises you perform, how many repetitions are done, and how much time was required. Most people find exercising to music enjoyable. Others find that watching TV or listening to the radio while exercising relieves boredom. The exercises can be done alone or with family or friends. Clothing should be loose, comfortable, and quite stretchable rather than restrictive. Shoes should have no heels and nonskid soles.

As we have previously discussed, your fitness program should ideally be completed in about 30 minutes. Once you can accomplish this, you are ready to substitute what may be more enjoyable and perhaps productive exercise pursuits. If you enjoy sports, then after your warm-up you may substitute on any given day 15 minutes of maximal exercise sports (running, stationary running, cycling, cross-country skiing, or swimming) (see Table 4-2), 30 minutes of moderate sports activity (tennis, skiing) (see Table 4-3) or 45 minutes of minimal exercise sports (golf, gardening, canoeing, bowling, fishing, archery, horseshoes, ping pong, shuffleboard, or social dancing) (see Table 4-4).

Just as sports can be graded into maximal, moderate, and minimal exercise and energy output, a number of household projects can also be graded and substituted for the exercise program. Some of these would include: in the maximal exercise group, chopping wood, shoveling snow, and digging holes; in the moderate group, mopping or scrubbing a floor, pushing a lawn mower, digging and pulling weeds; in the minimal exercise group, sweeping floors, ironing, washing clothes, making beds, and light gardening.

However, the single easiest way to increase physical activity is simply to walk whenever possible. Once you have attained level 1 fitness, then the elevator should be obsolete for fewer than three floors, and you should also be encouraged to park the car and walk at every chance.

Once you have successfully completed your fitness program in 30 minutes, you may substitute 30 to 60 minutes of any single or combined activity from Table 4-2, 60 to 90 minutes of activity from Table 4-3, or an hour or more of activity from Table 4-4.

The warm-up and cooling-off periods should not be forgotten when substituting other activities for the specific exercise routines. Five minutes of any exercise from pages 76–77 should precede your substituted activity, and 5 minutes of exercise from the same pages should follow it.

Inevitably, some people who have attained level 1 fitness will seek more vigorous endurance activity. Many men and women in their 60s and 70s have taken up jogging 2 or more miles daily. This is to be applauded; but do not substitute jogging for your entire exercise program. Although jogging is splendid cardiovascular exercise, it does nothing for upper-body muscle tone or joint flexibility and mobility. Jogging should always be preceded by stretching exercises and, in addition, calisthenics and other conditioning exercises listed in level 1 must be included if you are to achieve a balanced and complete workout.

After jogging, you should cool off with 5 minutes of walking or 5 minutes of exercises from pages 76–77.

Several additional points on jogging are especially pertinent to senior athletes. First, if you jog, you *must* wear appropriate running shoes. Basketball shoes, sneakers, or deck shoes will not suffice. Specially constructed running shoes provide foot and arch support and have multilayered, flat, nonskid soles that cushion the force of impact as you land on your feet. Unlike tennis shoes that do not have widths, good running shoes come in a variety of widths, and extreme care is essential in obtaining a precise fit. Most podiatrists recommend trying on shoes at the end of the day when your feet have swollen to their maximum size.

Second, when jogging wear soft loose-fitting clothing. Tight-fitting or abrasive clothing, heavy from perspiration, will chafe the skin, especially the nipples, groin, and armpits. It is seldom too cold to jog if you wear adequate clothing. This includes gloves and a hat or cap with adequate ear protection. Only a high wind chill factor should force you to exercise indoors, as jogging then may result in frostbite. Also, never jog on ice or other slippery surfaces.

Although it is rarely too cold to jog unless the wind chill factor is high, in the summer it is often too hot. Do not jog at midday, especially when temperatures and humidity are high. And replenish lost body fluids promptly either during or after your warm weather workout.

Nighttime jogging is also dangerous as you may stumble and fall. Only if a running area is adequately illuminated, like a lighted track, should you jog at night, and then only over known flat surfaces.

To conclude this chapter, let me mention two exercises that are nearly perfect for the total body—swimming and cross-country skiing. Unlike jogging, which does little to strengthen or increase upper body joint flexibility, they each combine a vigorous cardiovascular endurance workout with strengthening and increasing flexibility of nearly all joints. Both are highly recommended as an addition to your regular program.

Finally, let me state again the risks of competing in sports as opposed to following a personal fitness program. Competition should be avoided if the primary objective is physical fitness, because competition will invariably bring a stress-related injury resulting in an enforced layoff. However, for some—myself included—the stimulus of competition makes otherwise tedious exercise tolerable. Training that is not directed toward a specific objective is difficult to maintain. Also, there is a special joy in competing, whether against an opponent in tennis or against the clock in long-distance running. In distance races so many people usually enter that except for three or four in each class, the remainder are running against their previous best time. By retaining the common sense never to extend yourself too far in competition, its rewards will overshadow any minor injuries you may incur. However, no one should allow participation in one sport to replace his or her total exercise program.

Chapter 7

Female Athletes

"A horse perspires, a man sweats, but a woman just glows."

There is perhaps no domain where unfounded myths, attitudes, and beliefs remain so persistent as in the world of sports. Many of these misconceptions stem from the fact that sports, until very recently, were totally male orientated and dominated. In antiquity, the role of women in sports was discussed by Socrates in Plato's *Republic*. He raised the question whether "females should guard the flock and hunt with the males and take a share in all they do, or be kept within doors as fit for no more than bearing and feeding their children while all the hard work is left to the males." Socrates argued that both men and women ought to receive the same upbringing and education and that women should be given equal access to physical education. It only took about 2,400 years, until the Title IX legislation of 1974 that mandated women be included in all sports, for Socrates' views to be adopted. And as you know, although equality is mandated, it is incompletely funded.

In Greek antiquity, women were the "prize" of an athletic contest. Women could not compete in the Olympics, but they could own horses or a chariot; since prizes went to the owner and not the driver, some shared in victory. Only in Sparta were young women, separate from males, allowed to engage in physical activity.

During the Renaissance (1300–1600) in Italy, women of nobility were allowed to engage in sports activities. Humanists of that era believed physical activity could result in physical, moral, and even emotional well-being by raising the spirits and allaying depression.

In 1900 women were for the first time allowed to compete in the Olympics, which were held in Paris. They had been excluded from the first Olympic games in Athens in 1896. The reason women were allowed was that Pierre de Coubertin, founder of the modern Olympics and the most vociferous opponent of women in athletics, was demoted to a secondary role. Three years before his death in 1934, de Coubertin warned male athletes, "Contact with feminine athletes is bad" for it is "against the law of nature."

In the 1900 Olympics, women could compete only in tennis and golf. Archery was added in 1904, figure skating in 1908, swimming in 1912, and track and field in 1928. As recently as 1960, women competed in only 6 of 17 sports, and in 1976 only 50% of the competing countries sent women.

The old myth that women are too fragile to handle the emotional and physical demands of endurance sports has been shattered. Once excluded from the Olympic Games entirely, women now compete in the most grueling endurance event of all, the marathon. Since the Title IX legislation of 1974, there has been a more than 200% increase in the number of women competing in structured high school and college athletic programs. The improved performances of women clearly parallel established patterns observed in men.

Nonetheless, women differ from men in both anatomy and physiology, especially as regards different hormones and reproductive function. This chapter addresses the three major areas where exercise has unique influences on women as compared with men. They are: the effects of exercise on menstrual and reproductive function; special medical considerations, such as iron deficiency anemia; and unique musculoskeletal injury risks.

Effects of Exercise on Menstrual and Reproductive Function
Intense physical training has been shown in several studies to reduce the onset of puberty from 9 to 12 months. While many feel this is due to a reduction in body fat, the precise mechanism presently remains in dispute. Since long bones continue to grow until the completion of menarche (the first menstrual period), it also remains unclear whether this delay in puberty by physical training may result in increased height.

It is clear that many women undergoing intense training regimens experience a reduction in menstrual flow as well as numbers of periods. This also is thought to be tied to weight loss and low body fat content.

Presently it is clear that strenuous exercise may postpone the onset of menarche and may suppress or even, in extreme cases, cause a cessation in menses. There is no evidence, however, that it reduces fertility or future reproductive capacity once strenuous exercise is curtailed. Furthermore, for the conditioned female athlete, there is no indication that vigorous exercise is contraindicated even during the third trimester of pregnancy.

It appears that the benefits of being active for women include a reduced incidence of premenstrual tension, dysmenorrhea, and unusual menstrual conditions, such as toxic shock syndrome. The 1976 Montreal Olympic Games experience also clearly showed that menstruation does not exclude a world class performance, as gold medal winners performed during all phases of the menstrual cycle.

100

Medical Considerations

Women have a different body composition from men. In general, they have less muscle mass (23% of total body weight as compared with 40% in men) and more fat (22 to 25% is ideal for women, while 14 to 18% body fat is ideal for men). The muscle mass in the lower extremities is fairly equal for both sexes, but the amount of upper body muscle bulk is dramatically more in men. Since body fat is burned during endurance events such as marathon runs or swims, women may have an increased capacity for endurance training and performance. Future research will have to prove the validity of this hypothesis.

Anemia

Menstruation, with its obligatory iron loss, presents a potential risk for anemia. Several studies of healthy young college women have documented an incidence of mild anemia in up to 25% of those studied.

For endurance women athletes, care must be taken to distinguish between the pseudoanemia of endurance training and true anemia. When both men and women undertake a course of strenuous endurance training, their hemoglobin and red blood levels may fall, due to the effects of hemodilution as their total circulatory plasm volume is increased. Measurement of total iron stores as documented by normal serum iron and iron binding capacity and ferritin levels proves there is no true anemia. Thus, in both men and women endurance athletes, the establishment of true anemia requires the measurement of ferritin, serum iron, or iron binding capacity, and cannot be deduced from a random hematocrit or hemoglobin level.

Women, because of menstruation and slightly further iron loss in sweat, are at risk for true anemia. If present, even a mild anemia can have profound effects on performance in endurance events. If anemic, the endurance woman athlete cannot circulate as much oxygen to muscle and, thus, is operating under a severe handicap. An iron supplement can be given twice daily (300 mg ferrous sulfate tablets) for six months. It is important to realize that it usually takes at least half a year to fully replenish iron losses. Taking an iron supplement for a shorter period invites a recurrence of anemia. There is no evidence to suggest that excess iron is beneficial to performance. Thus, supplemental iron should not be taken unless true anemia is documented by low serum iron and iron binding capacity. The small amount of iron received from the common vitamins with iron is harmless for women, but it should not be taken by men who normally need no supplemental iron.

Environmental Stress

Even though there are obvious differences in body composition, women and men share identical cardiovascular and muscular patterns of response to endurance training, as well as adaptation to environmental stresses such as heat, cold, and altitude. Acclimatization to hot weather is facilitated by

Table 7-1
Common Athletic Injuries According to Sex

Women	Men
Tibial stress syndrome (runners)	Achilles peritendinitis (runners)
Lower-extremity injuries (cross-country skiers)	Patellofemoral pain syndrome (runners)
Recurrent patellar subluxation	Knee injuries in general (runners)
Tibial and femoral stress fractures and overuse injuries (all sports)	Overexertion injuries in fit middle-aged men (all sports)
Stress-related injuries such as sprains, strains, and heat illness (all sports)	Iliotibial friction band syndrome

*Reproduced with permission from *Sports Medicine in Primary Care* by Robert C. Cantu, M.D., © 1982 D.C. Heath and Company.

underlying fitness, but still requires 7 to 10 days for optimal adaptation. Whether it be heat acclimatization or adaptation to cold or altitude, the considerations appear identical for women and men endurance athletes.

Musculoskeletal Injuries

The female anatomy, in addition to the obvious external sexual differences from men, includes a wider pelvis, which places additional stress on the knees. This results in an increased incidence of patellar syndromes. Thus, women undertaking sports that primarily use the lower extremities (e.g., running, soccer, rugby) should exercise extra caution during the initial weeks of training. A prolonged warm-up plus leg flexibility and muscle strengthening exercises may ease the musculoskeletal stress during this initial high-risk period. Women should pay special attention to a very gradual increase in training to avoid overuse syndromes. It is also prudent to have footwear, to avoid unidirectional running on hard or uneven surfaces, and to pay attention to external training factors (heat, cold, altitude) that influence injury rates. If injured, the treatment of musculoskeletal injuries in women is the same as for men. Table 7-1 depicts the most common injuries in female and male athletes. Sprains and strains account for most of the injuries in female athletes. This can be explained by the fact that women have valgus knees, more body fat than men, greater joint mobility, more elastic connective tissue, smaller tendons, and less stabilizing muscle mass. Basketball, field hockey, gymnastics, and volleyball are responsible for most women's sports injuries. The breast, contrary to a popular misconception, is rarely injured in women's sports. Equally untrue is the belief that vigorous exercise may lead to sagging of the breasts or wrinkles on the face, and that vigorous running in women contributes to varicose veins or uterine prolapse.

Chapter 8

Obese Athletes

All of us who are seriously committed to a total physical fitness program must also think seriously about and strive to achieve near optimum body weight. Obesity in the United States rises rapidly at age 25, and by the fifth decade of life, one-third of American men and over half of American women are more than 20% overweight (obese). Today society views obesity as distinctly undesirable. Since the turn of the century, slenderness has been the ideal. Professional models and beauty contest winners are no longer overweight.

Most Americans now believe obesity is the number one nutrition problem, a condition of "caloric excess." People of the twentieth century do not like to be fat. They dislike the stigma of obesity. The concept of the "jolly" fat man or woman is pure myth. Most obese people agonize over walking appreciable distances, getting into a small car, or even buying clothes. In fact, hostility has been shown to be a key behavior reaction among obese people. Over 50 million Americans spend over $100 million annually for a quick, easy way to lose weight. If one includes dietetic foods, "fat mills," "health spas," appetite-suppressing drugs, special exercise equipment, and the numerous devices for alleged spot fat loss, the monetary figure zooms to over $10 billion in the United States alone.

To be obese places a severe strain on your body, and the strain is even greater while exercising. That is why I have selected out specific exercise programs for obese people. More important, obesity contributes directly to hypertension and adult onset diabetes (70 to 80% of maturity onset diabetics are obese) and indirectly to heart disease and stroke. Life insurance companies' statistics clearly show that the overall death rate of the obese adult is more than 50% greater than that of the normal weight adult of comparable age.

High blood pressure and obesity have both been identified as risk factors for coronary heart disease. Hypertension also increases the chance of stroke and accelerates the process of atherosclerosis. It has been shown that as people gain weight, they experience proportionally higher levels of blood pressure (hypertension) and cardiovascular disease. These patterns appear in both sexes, but are more prominent in men. For example, middle-aged men who are 30% overweight are four times more likely to die suddenly of heart attack and seven times more likely to suffer a stroke than are lean males of comparable age.

While research during the past 10 years has established a direct relationship between obesity and hypertension, it has been shown that a fall in blood pressure can be expected with a reduction in weight. A 15% drop in weight in men is associated with a 10% drop in blood pressure. The same is true for women; thus, weight control is a potent tool in the control of hypertension in overweight subjects. In fact, weight reduction should be recommended as the initial step in the treatment of any hypertensive patient who is above ideal weight.

Obesity has also been linked to elevated blood cholesterol levels. However, the effect of obesity on blood pressure is considerably greater than on cholesterol. Obesity is dangerous primarily because it causes hypertension. Now, most physicians recommend caloric restriction as the treatment of choice for the mildly hypertensive overweight patient. Actually, the best treatment is one of combined exercise and diet, esepecially since tests have established that strenuous, regular exercise by itself usually results in some weight loss and a lowering of blood pressure.

Unfortunately, our understanding of the relationship between diet and exercise and a reduction in weight and blood pressure is still tentative. How obesity predisposes to hypertension, for example, is as unclear as how it is associated with diabetes. In view of the great number of obese hypertensive people in our society, the federal government should deal with this serious problem by making and funding an intensive research commitment in this area of health care.

What Constitutes Obesity and How Is It Measured?

It is essential to realize that being overweight and being obese are not necessarily synonymous, even though in practical terms obese generally means more than 15 to 20% overweight. Realistically, obesity should be regarded as 15% or more excess body fat. Overweight refers to weight in excess of normal as compared with sex, height, and body-frame weight tables. It includes all body components including muscle, water, minerals, and tissue, as well as fat. Thus, weight lifters and body builders who have markedly enhanced muscle development may be grossly "overweight," but they may have no excess fat and thus not be obese. The basic concept exists, then, that obesity refers only to body fat, the tissue accumulated exclusively by caloric excess. Body fat can be measured by several techniques as discussed in Chapter 3.

Why We Become Obese and How To Correct It

While rare hypothalamic, genetic, and drug-induced obesities do occur, almost all adult onset obesity is simply due to the fact that more calories are consumed than are used by the body. The elimination of obesity requires decreasing caloric intake, increasing caloric expenditure, or preferably both so that, until a desirable weight is achieved, the body runs a daily deficit of calories and burns body fat to compensate.

As discussed in the nutrition chapter, over a long period of time, the composition of the diet (if nutritionally adequate) really doesn't matter, as long as there is a deficit of calories. Although many studies have shown that the most precipitous weight loss on a short-term diet occurs with a high-fat diet, the next greatest weight loss with a high-protein diet, and least weight loss with a high-carbohydrate diet, the impressive rapid drop in weight on the high-fat diet reflects water loss and not fat reduction. This is analogous to jogging in a rubber suit to enhance perspiring and, thus, rapidly depleting body water and, temporarily, body weight. Given access to fluids, the depleted body water will eventually be replaced, and only the true fat loss, about a deficit of 3500 kcal per pound, will be reflected on the scales.

The Analogy Between Obesity and Diabetes

It is now clear that overcoming obesity requires a reduction in caloric intake below caloric expenditure. You must: (1) determine where you are out of caloric balance (overeating, inactivity, or both); (2) recognize "problem" times of the day and associated activities; (3) encourage small but well-reinforced changes (i.e., ones that are likely to be permanent such as extra walking rather than jogging at 5 a.m.); (4) encourage no more than 1 or 2 pounds of weight loss per week, which calculates out to a 500-calorie deficient diet each day; (5) discourage fad diets and emphasize a nutritious diet around natural food preferences; and (6) encourage eating slowly by setting down utensils between mouthfuls and chewing well so you will feel satiated with less food.

In addition, there must be a lucid plan of weight maintenance once the desired weight is achieved. Most now feel the weight maintenance phase should be simultaneous with the weight loss phase. It should be pictured as an ongoing process, because there are no known cures for adult onset obesity except caloric equilibrium. Here, there is a strong parallel with diabetes. In any illness, while a physician accepts the responsibility for the initial diagnosis and treatment plan, the ultimate day-to-day management of the condition is up to you, the patient. Whereas the weight loss phase may be under the direction of a physician, the success of the weight maintenance phase rests with you.

Inherent in weight maintenance is education in a nutritionally adequate, appetite-satisfying, low-to-moderate calorie diet. While personal preferences must be taken into consideration, some general features include the following:

1. Lean meat, fish, or fowl at least once daily, plus up to three eggs weekly.

2. Unsweetened cereal or a slice of whole wheat bread two or three times daily.

3. Green or yellow vegetables twice daily.

4. Fruit or fruit juice twice daily.

5. Consume at least 300 calories at each of three of four meals without snacking.

6. Take reasonable size portions without second servings.

7. Broil, boil, bake, or roast meat and fish; remove visible fat; avoid thickened gravy.

8. Cook vegetables without fat; flavor with vegetable margarine, herbs, or bouillon.

9. Favor green, yellow, or red vegetables over starchy ones.

10. On salads, use low-calorie dressings, lemon juice, or vinegar.

11. Favor plain fruit over pastries for dessert.

12. Sweeten with sugar substitutes; use only sugar-free soft drinks.

13. Eat meals at about the same time each day with regular intervals in between.

14. Favor nonfat milk and ice milk or low-fat ice cream.

15. Minimize alcoholic beverages; use "lite" beers; use sugar-free soft drinks as mixers.

An Exercise Program Tailored To Obese People

While obese people can lose weight with diet alone, diet reduction and especially maintenance is far easier and more successful when a program of exercise is simultaneously employed. Exercise not only burns up calories, but it also can act as an appetite suppressant. An appropriate exercise program, while important for anyone because of the many physical and psychological benefits, acquires an even more cogent significance for obese people. This is because such a program combats the various risk factors of cardiovascular disease and stroke that obesity promotes—diabetes, hypertension, and hyperlipidemia.

An appropriate exercise program for obese people shares most of the same basic features as one for the less plump, that is, a warm-up period, an aerobic endurance phase, and a cooling-off period. The frequency of exercise should not be less than three days per week, and preferably should be more. Before it is commenced, however, a medical examination and probably a stress electrocardiogram should be obtained, because of the greater risk of heart disease in obese people.

The warm-up and cooling-off periods should last 5 to 10 minutes. Each involves rhythmic slow stretching movements of the trunk and limbs that emphasize range of motion of joints. Carried out before vigorous exercise, these movements enhance blood flow and stretch and loosen one's muscles, preparing them for sustained activity and minimizing the chance for strains or sprains. Following vigorous exertion, these movements facilitate the various bodily functions' gradual return to normal and promote the elimination of waste products from your muscles, thereby lessening the possibility of stiffness or soreness the following day. Calisthenics are ideal for each of these periods. On pages 76 and 77 you can find specific exercises for each of these periods listed. You may select any combination of three or more from each table to constitute your own warm-up and cooling-off periods. It is recommended that you vary the selection of exercises on different days, both to avoid monotony and to ensure total body involvement.

The most important portion of your exercise program as regards weight reduction and all the other gains discussed in Chapter 1 is the endurance phase. This phase should ideally involve activities that use the large muscle groups of the body in a continuous, rhythmic, aerobic manner. The duration should eventually exceed 30 minutes, although a more modest beginning may be necessary. As the training effect is realized and your aerobic capacity is enhanced, you may increase the intensity and duration of this period. It is never recommended for purposes of attaining fitness that you exceed an intensity greater than 60 to 80% of your maximal oxygen uptake or heart rate (about 120–140 beats per minute), nor a duration of 1 hour. While competitive athletes must exceed these limits in order to achieve maximum performance, it is done so at a significantly increased risk of injury. This risk of injury is unacceptable to your exercise program, so while enthusiasm is to be applauded, avoid getting "carried away."

In the upright position, the excess weight of obesity places greater stresses especially on your low back, hips, knees, ankles, and feet, both at rest and even more so with exertion. Thus, the types of endurance exercises best suited for obese people are more restricted than for slender people. In Table 8-1 some of the better endurance exercises for obese people are listed. Jogging or running are not included because the strain on the low back and lower extremities is too great. An increased incidence of injury of up to 50% can be anticipated for an obese person who begins a jogging program. Clearly, activities involving running and jumping, where obesity accentuates the vertical stresses to the musculoskeletal system, are to be avoided.

If you are "temporarily" obese, the best pursuits are those done either in the water (body surfing, scuba diving, skin diving, swimming, or water polo), those pursued in a sitting position (bicycling, canoeing, kayaking, and rowing), or those done erect without much running or jumping (backpacking, boxing, cross-country skiing, handball, hiking, ice hockey, ice-skating, karate, racquet ball, roller-skating, snowshoeing, squash, walking, and wrestling).

Swimming is the best all-around aerobic exercise for obese people, because all the major muscle groups receive vigorous exercise, while the stresses to the skeletal system of the body are minimal and are actually

Table 8-1
Aerobic Endurances Exercise Pursuits for Obese People

Backpacking	Paddle ball
Bicycling	Racquet ball
Body surfing	Roller-skating
Boxing	Rowing
Canoeing	Scuba diving
Cross-country skiing	Skin diving
Handball	Snowshoeing
Hiking	Squash
Ice hockey	Swimming
Ice-skating	Walking
Karate	Wrestling
Kayaking	Water polo

made less by the increased body fat. Body fat adds to one's buoyancy in water and partially accounts for the fact that most great marathon swimmers are on the chubby side. Swimming is also rhythmic, by definition continuous, and of necessity aerobic. Thus, it meets all the criteria of a good endurance exercise without allowing the excess weight to stress one's skeletal system.

However, after you have shed weight by the combination of diet and your own exercise program, I encourage you to explore the additional exercises found in Chapter 4. With a diligent approach, your obesity will be temporary, and as you enter the weight maintenance phase that we all must pursue for the rest of our lives, only personal preferences need limit your choice of recreational pursuits.

Chapter 9

Medical Problems Caused By Exercise

There are a number of real medical problems and some not so real medical conditions arising from exercise. Included in the latter category are heart enlargement seen in endurance athletes, pseudoanemia due to increased plasma volume, and abnormal urinary sediment, which suggests kidney disease but is due rather to volume depletion as a result of exhaustive exercise. This chapter deals with those real and apparently real conditions observed in competitive and recreational athletes.

Anaphylaxis

Anaphylaxis is an allergic condition that begins with diffuse itching but may progress to generalized hives, facial swelling, and potentially fatal swelling and spasm of the upper airway plus a low blood pressure. It is the same type of allergic reaction that some susceptible people have to a bee sting or to ingestion of certain shellfish. A type of blood cell called a mast cell releases substances including histamine, bradykinins, and other mediators that produced the generalized swelling and vascular collapse.

Exercise-induced anaphylaxis usually occurs in people with a history of allergic reactions such as childhood exema, seasonal rhinitis, or asthma. Incredible as it may seem, symptoms may first occur suddenly after years of exercise without symptoms. The condition is not related to training or degree of fitness; it strikes world record–holders and weekend athletes alike. The precise cause is not clearly known, but some feel that an exposure to a specific allergen, such as shellfish to which one is subclinically allergic, when combined with exercise may precipitate the full-blown reaction.

Treatment of this condition may include taking a mild antihistamine or sodium chromalin, or avoiding specific foods prior to exercise. If a severe attack occurs, one should immediately stop exercising, self-administer 0.1 to 0.3 ml of 1:1000 epinephrine into the fat beneath the skin if you have such a syringe, and be taken to your hospital emergency room. Fortunately, unlike anaphylactic reactions to bee stings and shellfish, which may prove fatal, there have to date been no reports of fatality with exercise-induced anaphylaxis. Nonetheless, it is not a condition to be taken lightly. If it has occurred, it would be prudent to exercise with a loaded epinephrine syring as a close companion. You can purchase one at a drug store with a doctor's prescription.

Asthma

As is true for exercise-induced anaphylaxis, exercise-provoked asthma also occurs in individuals with an allergic background, especially for asthma itself.

Asthma is a spasm of the bronchioles, your smaller lung air passages. It typically occurs after a slow buildup, 6 to 8 minutes into vigorous exercise. In some, the attack may stabilize or lessen, allowing you to exercise through the attack. Others will have to reduce the severity of the exercise. There also may be a recurrence of the attack after exercise has ceased in those who have been able to exercise through the attack. It also appears that the cooler the air and the lower the humidity, the more likely an attack is to occur. This explains why some runners only experience this condition in the winter and can eliminate it by breathing warmer, inspired air. Some ingenious runners with this condition during the winter run a hose from under their shirt or coat to a mask in front of their face, thus affording themselves warm, moist air to breathe.

Other treatments include the standard medications, such as bronchodilators (sodium chromalin), traditionally used to treat asthma. A slow, progressive warm-up period may also attenuate the reaction. Many inhalers use adrenalin compounds that are not allowed in many formal competitive situations. Fortunately, sodium chromalin is acceptable, even in the Olympics.

Finally, rather than be discouraged, those susceptible to exercise-induced asthma should be encouraged to participate in sports. Only by so doing will they achieve the beneficial effects of general physical conditioning, plus the maximal preservation of lung function. Despite the need for specific protective measures or medication, such individuals are urged to lead full, active athletic lives.

Environmental Factors

Altitude, cold, and heat are environmental factors that present special hazards to world class and recreational athletes alike. Clearly, prevention is the best medicine, and this section will be devoted to imparting such information.

Cold weather endurance exertion poses the major danger of fatigue resulting in decreased work effort, leading to a fall in body temperature due to environmental losses. Wind speed affects the wind-chill factor, which essentially lowers the effective temperature. It is possible to lower body temperatures to a point that heart arrhythmias or arrest may result. Prolonged strenuous exertion without adequate heat dissipation from overdressing or wearing materials that do not breathe may lead to volume depletion, in spite of cold conditions, although this happens infrequently.

Rapid warming is the treatment of mild to moderate reductions in body temperature (hypothermia). In cold weather, it is wise to wear a hat, as the scalp is a major source of heat loss. Your ear lobes and nose also should be covered. Although significant discomfort may be experienced when forcefully breathing cold air, frostbite of the lungs or airways does not occur.

Heat injury poses a life-threatening risk to endurance athletes. It spans a spectrum from heat exhaustion, with rectal temperatures under 40°C, to the potentially fatal stroke with body temperatures in excess of 41°C. Heat injury involves a number of factors, including the state of the athlete's conditioning, perceived level of exertion, temperature, humidity, and sunshine. Metabolic heat is produced by exercise and dissipated primarily by sweating. One mile of running would produce a 3°F elevation in your body temperature, if the heat were not lost. Solar radiation (sunshine), air temperature, humidity, and movement all affect the rate at which your body heat can be dissipated. As humidity rises, less sweat can evaporate and dissipate heat; thus, higher temperatures become even more hazardous. Direct sunlight further enhances this risk.

Preventive measures include starting hot weather endurance exercise with extra fluid intake equal to anticipated losses. Fluids should also be consumed liberally during the event; but since absorption from the stomach during vigorous exercise is much reduced, the key is starting in an over-hydrated state. Clothing should be loose and light. If sun cannot be avoided, a cap should be worn to shade the head. Another important factor is acclimatization, which increases the rate of sweating and reduces sodium sweat losses.

While heat stress certainly is more common in inexperienced endurance athletes who cannot adequately monitor their exertional levels, even world class athletes are not exempt from heat stress. Alberto Salizar, the current world record holder for the marathon in 1979, collapsed while in first place within one-half mile of the finish line of a 7.3-mile race in Falmouth, Mass. He was given the last rites and taken to a local hospital with a temperature in excess of 41°C, but fortunately recovered.

The main symptoms of heat injury are abdominal cramps and nausea, followed by dizziness and confusion. While diminished sweating may still occur, chills may also be experienced. The loss of blood volume leads to a rapid pulse and low blood pressure. Athletes who perceive these symptoms during an endurance event should stop and immediately drink cool fluids while cooling off. Immediate rapid cooling on-site without delay is the ideal treatment of heat injury. Delay may lead to fatal kidney, liver, or blood clotting problems.

Heart

Sudden death does occur in athletes. When it occurs in the teens, twenties, or early thirties, it is usually due to inherited congenital heart abnormalities, especially of the heart muscle itself. The usual story is that of a high school, college, or young adult athlete who suddenly "drops dead" while vigorously exercising either in a game or in practice. While his coaches and peers will almost always state they thought he was in vigorous good health, it is common for there to be a family history of sudden death and a personal previous history of sudden fainting for no apparent reason. A physical examination may reveal high blood pressure or abnormal heart murmurs, and an electrocardiogram often shows abnormalities consistent with unequal cardiac muscle enlargement. While this is exceedingly tragic when it occurs, it is fortunately rare. Since it would cost more than $150 to evaluate each athlete in depth to rule out such inherited disorders, it is not practical to do so. However, if you have a family history of sudden death or have "blacked out" for no apparent reason, it would be prudent to undergo a thorough cardiac evaluation. While such individuals may certainly not anticipate a normal life expectancy, it clearly can be lengthened by avoidance of vigorous exercise.

Sudden death may also occur in athletes over 40. While this may sometimes be due to less severe inherited heart muscle abnormalities are previously discussed, it is most frequently the result of coronary artery heart disease. Rather extensive coronary artery atherosclerosis has been shown in some endurance athletes, including marathon runners. While beneficial, strenuous exercise is no guarantee against heart attack. Thus, individuals over 40 who are embarking on vigorous exercise programs and who have recognized risk factors for heart attack (a family history of heart disease, personal history of hypertension, hypercholesterolemia, or cigarette smoking) are encouraged to undergo a stress electrocardiogram. For those over 40 who are already vigorously exercising without risk factors or any cardiac symptoms, such as shortness of breath, chest pain, or fainting, stress testing is unnecessary.

I believe it is important for all of us to reflect on the fact that although an active life-style, including moderate amounts of vigorous exercise, does promote cardiovascular fitness and a reduced risk of heart attack, it does not convey immortality or guarantee that you will never have a heart attack. Furthermore, sustained activity for 30 minutes three to four times a week is all that is required. Excessive physical exertion, such as long-distance running and marathon competition, may well carry additional risks for the heart without further protective benefits. To best facilitate and preserve health, we should seek a life-style with a balanced approach to exercise, diet, and alcohol.

Before concluding comments about the heart and exercise, it is important to discuss heart muscle changes in response to exercise. Depending on the type of exercise, the heart may change in muscle mass, chamber size, or both. Endurance athletes tend to have dilated chambers, especially the left ventricle, which also develops a slightly thicker wall. On the other hand, weight lifters with their isometric strength training develop an increase in total heart muscle without any chamber enlargement. The heart of the endurance athlete has adapted to handle a high-volume flow of blood, an increased volume pumping ability. The heart of the strength athlete changes to be able to pump the same amount of blood against a much greater resistance. It is important to realize that this enlargement is a natural accompaniment of exercise. Thus, for the athlete without heart symptoms (chest pain or sudden fainting), an enlarged heart with expected electrocardiogram abnormalities does not require the provocative or invasive heart testing that would be recommended in the nonathlete suspected of having heart disease.

Psychological Factors

Exercise can exert a profound effect on your total health and well-being. It can alter not only your body composition and capacity, but your psychological makeup as well. Lately a great deal has been written about the positive addiction of regular endurance exercise. While there is still no real proof of a "runner's high," there is a great deal of evidence to substantiate the fact that regular exercise results in a better self-image and a positive outlook. It is now being used to treat depression and anxiety states. There is no hard evidence to suggest that regular exercise will change your personality type from a hard-driving, compulsive Type A to a more relaxed, laid-back Type B. There is also no evidence to confirm it will heighten your sexual capacity, either in performance or enjoyment. There is, however, plenty of evidence that those who suddenly undertake an obsessive, unchecked extreme commitment to exercise risk disruption of vital personal ties, both at work and in the family. Divorce is higher in overcommitted recreational runners, such as those entering marathons, than in society at large. This again points out another reason for the admonition for regular endurance exercise, but in moderation.

Urology

In contrast to contact sports, where blood in the urine may reflect a traumatic kidney blood clot and warrants a thorough evaluation including intravenous pyelography (IVP), endurance exertion may produce harmless asymptomatic blood in the urine. If there is significant volume depletion (dehydration), protein sediment may also be found in the urine. Thus, the presence of blood or protein after extreme endurance exertion is not un-expected and need not trigger a visit to your urologist or family physician. Obviously, the presence of blood in the urine on successive days or not after extreme exercise could not be explained by this mechanism, and a call to your doctor is in order.

Muscle tissue is broken down by extreme endurance exercise resulting in the muscle pigment (myoglobin) appearing in urine and serum muscle enzymes (serum creatine kinase) being elevated up to 30 times.

The most serious kidney injury occurs with severe dehydration (as in heat stress injury) and involves damage to the kidney cells. This can rarely lead to kidney failure and even death. It is entirely preventable by adequate hydration. Thus, again the caution to start an endurance event with an excess of fluids equal to anticipated losses, consume fluids liberally during the event, and immediately rehydrate at the conclusion. This rehydration should be sufficient to allow you to produce the golden flow. It is a sign of possibly serious renal injury if you cannot void within several hours of rehydrating after an endurance event.

Section III

Sports Injuries: Prevention, Treatment, And Rehabilitation

Chapter 10

An Overview

The next six chapters are devoted to a discussion of sports injury prevention, treatment, and rehabilitation, with regard to both the various areas of your body and their relative risk of injury depending on the sport you are playing. We will stress the contribution of errors in technique and improper training or equipment to sports injuries, and we will discuss appropriate protective equipment. This will lead us to the final two chapters in which personal conditioning programs will be outlined for each of the common recreational pursuits and my personal mythical ranking of the top ten sports will be discussed, taking into consideration accessibility, cost, degree of aerobic fitness, degree of total body exercise, and safety.

However, before we dissect each injury by sport and area of the body, I believe it is appropriate for you to know some of the terminology of sports injuries and to be aware of the most frequent injuries seen at sports medicine clinics, the sports that produced them, and some general principles of initial treatment and rehabilitation.

Microtrauma versus Macrotrauma

There are two ways in which you may incur a sports injury. The first is by a single episode of high-impact (macro) trauma, as by a blow or a fall. The second is from many repetitive episodes of lesser trauma (repetitive microtrauma), as in tennis elbow or running injuries. We adult recreational athletes often neglect overall general conditioning, systematic training, and proper warm-up, making us especially prone to this second type of injury, which is often referred to as a stress or overuse injury.

Bone Injuries

The most common injuries involve bone, cartilage, ligaments, muscle-tendon units, or the skin. Bone injuries involve either a bruise with swelling and tenderness or a fracture or break. Diagnostic x-rays or bone scans document the fracture, as in the case of stress fractures from repetitive activity, such as running or jumping. Pain alone or in combination with swelling may be the only symptom and sign of a stress fracture, which often is initially misdiagnosed as tendinitis. Most stress fractures are the result of improper training—usually too much and too intense training over too short a time. Improper footwear or a minor bone, joint, or muscle imbalance may contribute to an injury. Cortisone injections and anti-inflammatory drugs (aspirin, Butazoladin, Clinoril, Indocin, Motrin, Tolectin) may partially mask the pain. If you persist in training despite constant pain, a stress fracture may progress to complete displacement. Often invisible on regular x-rays, a stress fracture may best be identified with a bone scan.

Cartilage Injury

A joint consists of two articulating bones. The surface where the bones actually touch is covered with articular cartilage. The most common diagnosis in most sports medicine clinics is chondromalacia patella, a degeneration and roughening of the articular cartilage of the kneecap (patella). Often due to improper tracking or movement of the patella, it is usually correctable with quadricep muscle strengthening exercises as discussed in Chapter 15.

Ligament Injury (Sprain)

Ligaments are connective tissue that unite bones and, thus, stabilize the bones of a joint. A sprain occurs when a ligament is stressed beyond its normal capabilities, causing it to stretch or tear. Sprains usually result from a single episode of macrotrauma and, depending on the extent of ligamentous damage and resultant joint instability, are classified as first-, second-, or third-degree sprains. There is tenderness and swelling over the ligament, but the joint is stable, and little functional impairment is present in a first-degree sprain. In addition to greater tenderness and swelling, there is some joint instability, but not enough to eliminate satisfactory joint function in a second-degree sprain. In a third-degree sprain, there is complete disruption of the ligament with resultant gross instability of the joint on the side of the ruptured ligament.

Sprains are the most common athletic injury, usually occurring at hinged joints (ankle, knee, finger). The immediate treatment of a sprain is the same regardless of degree. The acronym RICE stands for the four steps in treatment.

1) Rest: This allows torn blood vessels to contract and coagulate, minimizing further tissue injury and swelling.

2) Ice: Intermittent 5- to 10-minute periods of the application of ice

reduces swelling and minimizes bleeding. Chemical coolant bags usually have a short period of cooling and may cause skin burns if they leak.

3) Compression: A compression wrap, most easily provided by gentle elastic wraps, further retards swelling, bleeding, and joint effusion.

4) Elevation: In order to ensure drainage and blood return, the injured area should be elevated above the heart.

This initial treatment of sprains has traditionally been carried out for 24 to 48 hours. Recent experience suggests it may be benficial for 5 to 7 days. Hypothermia, because of its anti-inflammatory and analgesic effects, appears to aid recovery and early rehabilitation.

The second stage of treatment involves the progressive return of motion of the affected joints by rehabilitative exercises. Local heat is helpful in relaxing muscles and enhancing the flow of blood to the area. The exercise may be either isometric or dynamic, but must be done without pain or recurrent swelling, which indicate that the healing limits are being exceeded and a delay in the healing process is being risked.

The final stage in recovery from injury is the restoration of complete strength and range of motion. Since stretched ligaments do not possess the complete capacity to retighten themselves, it involves primarily the strengthening of muscles around a joint that will aid in its stabilization, keeping it strong so that reinjury can be avoided.

While a ligament attaches one bone to another, a tendon attaches a muscle to bone. Muscles can be likened to motorized rubber bands. Muscles have the capacity both to be stretched and to contract, exerting forces across a joint. Most recreational sports place demands on both the strength and flexibility of muscles. Many recreational athletes strengthen muscles, but fail to concentrate equally on flexibility and incur injuries stemming from the lack of flexibility of muscle groups.

Muscle-Tendon Injury (Strain)

Tears of either the muscle or its tendinous insertion are referred to as strains. They occur from either a simple explosive episode of macrotrauma or repeated microtrauma (overuse). Strains are graded from 1 to 3 (gross disruption of a muscle or its tendon) according to the same criteria discussed for sprains.

Most strains are self-induced and do not involve external forces. Muscolutendinous elasticity diminishes with age, making our tendons weaker. This makes the warm-up with proper stretching mandatory for adults.

Treatment of strains involves the same initial therapy (RICE) and second- and final-stage therapy as discussed for sprains. The most precise measurement of muscle strength, power, and endurance is today available by using the Cybex Isokinetic Dynamometer. Final recovery of a strain has not occurred until measurements of performance on the Cybex are equal for an injured and uninjured limb and muscle bulk has been restored.

Site of Injury and Sport Responsible

Tables 10-1 and 10-2 reflect a 4-year experience with more than a thousand patients at a large sports medicine clinic in New York City. A similar experience has been seen at the Children's Hospital Medical Center Division of Sports Medicine in Boston.

It is important to keep in mind that the injuries seen at a sports medicine clinic are generally more serious or refractory to treatment. By this I mean that many of the mild sprains and strains are handled by a trainer or school

Table 10-1
Injury By Anatomic Site

Location	%
Knee	46
Ankle	10
Shoulder	8
Foot	7
Elbow	6
Back	5
Hip	5
Tibia	4
Other	9

Table 10-2
Sport Responsible For Injury

Sport	%
Running-jogging	35
Racquet sports	12
Basketball	11
Ballet/dancing	7
Football	4
Snow skiing	4
Weight lifting	3
Baseball/softball	3
Martial arts	3
Other	18

physician or by recreational athletes themselves. Referral to a clinic is usually made only if the injury is thought to be more serious or does not respond to initial treatment. Thus, the most common sports injury, a sprain of the lateral ligaments of the ankle, is not the injury seen most often in sports medicine clinics, because it usually never reaches a doctor's care. This injury is most frequently incurred by cutting runs, as in football or soccer, or landing improperly (often on someone else's foot) after a jump, say in basketball or aerobic dance. So, too, serious head, face, and cervical spine injuries do not make their appearances at sports medicine clinics, because they are directly taken care of by neurosurgical and maxillofacial surgeons. Sports medicine clinics are largely staffed by orthopedists, podiatrists, and physical therapists, who are most skilled in treating bone, cartilage, ligament, and muscle injuries. Thus, with these referral patterns in mind, let's look at the sports medicine clinic experience.

Whether it be New York or Boston, the knee is by far the most common joint injured, running-jogging is the most common source of injury, and the kneecap (patella) is the portion of the knee most injured. Undoubtedly it is the recent explosion in the numbers of adults participating in long-distance running (estimated to be nearing 40 million) that accounts for running being the leading cause of injury. The ankle, shoulder, foot, and elbow are the next most often injured areas of the body with racquet sports, basketball, and dancing being the responsible activity. After kneecap disorders, strains, skeletal (bone) injuries, and sprains are the next most common diagnoses.

I have now briefly discussed the most common injury terminology, the site and diagnosis of injuries, and the sport of origin. In the next five chapters, we will look in depth at the most common injuries and how they can be prevented by proper training and technique as well as by using protective equipment.

Chapter 11

Head, Face, Eye, and Mouth Injuries

The central nervous system (brain, retina of the eye, and spinal cord) is unique in that nerve cells are not capable of regeneration. Injury to these structures takes on a singular importance, since cells that die are forever lost. While virtually every major joint (ankle, knee, hip, elbow, shoulder) and most of the body's organs can be replaced, the central nervous system is not capable of regrowth, transplantation, or replacement with artificial hardware. With these sobering facts in mind, it is quite obvious why prevention, rather than rehabilitation, is the key with head and facial injuries. Also, it is obvious that brain, eye, and mouth injuries require immediate medical attention, since self-treatment can result in loss of sight or even life itself. In fact, most head, eye, mouth, and face injuries are even beyond the competence of the primary care physician to evaluate and treat. Referral to a neurosurgeon or dental, oral, plastic, or eye surgeon is appropriate. For this reason (unlike the next four chapters, which will have roughly equal emphasis on prevention, treatment, and rehabilitation), in this chapter injury recognition and prevention, especially as regards protective equipment and proper technique, will be stressed. Table 11-1 ranks some common recreational pursuits with regard to risk of head, eye, face, and mouth injury.

Head Injuries

Concussion
The most common athletic brain injury is concussion. While this is physiologically defined as a transient alteration of brain function (usually with a period of unconsciousness) followed by complete brain recovery,

123

Table 11-1

| | Injury to | | |
Head	Eye	Face	Mouth
Archery	L	L	L	L
Automobile racing	H	M	M	M
Baseball	M	M	M	M
Basketball	L	M	M	M
Bicycling	M	M	L	L
Bowling	L	L	L	L
Diving	L	L	L	L
Football	H	L	L	L
Golf	L	L	L	L
Gymnastics	L	L	L	L
Handball	L	H	M	M
Hang gliding	H	M	M	M
Ice hockey	H	L*	L*	L*
Ice-skating	M	L	L	L
Lacrosse	H	L	L	L
Motorcycle racing	H	H	H	H
Racquetball	L	H	M	M
Roller-skating	M	L	M	M
Rowing	L	L	L	L
Rugby	M	M	H	M
Running	L	L	L	L
Skiing	M	L	L	L
Soccer	M	L	M	M
Squash	L	H	M	M
Swimming	L	L	L	L
Tennis	L	H	L	L
Volleyball	M	L	L	L
Water skiing	M	L	L	L
Weight lifting	L	L	L	L
Wrestling				

L = low risk of injury   M = moderate risk of injury   H = high risk of injury   L* = low risk of injury with full face mask, otherwise high

many concussions occur without a lapse in consciousness. This has led to a clinical grading of concussions. In the most mild form (grade I), there is no loss of consciousness, but only lapse of memory after the head trauma. Many boxers have instinctively won fights after blows to the head rendered them amnesic for events following an early round. (I will have more to say about boxing later.) Also, it is not uncommon for a football player to "have his bell rung" during a given play and then to play the rest of the game without subsequently being able to recall it.

In the more severe grades of concussion, you are unconscious transiently (grade II) or for a more prolonged time (grade III). In this instance, the head trauma causes alterations in the function of the reticular activating system that runs from the upper cervical spinal cord to the thalamus, resulting in unconsciousness and associated changes in pulse, respiration, and blood pressure. Consciousness, motor power, and coordination are regained as the reticular activating system resumes normal function.

Generally speaking, the degree and duration of amnesia correlates with the severity of the concussion. In grade I, your amnesia is usually only for events immediately after the head trauma (retrograde amnesia). But in grade III, events preceding the trauma may also be lost (anterograde amnesia). For student or recreational athletes, a grade II or III concussion requires that they be removed from the game, that they obtain skull x-rays, and that they stay in a medical facility for 24 hours of neurologic observation. With a grade I concussion, in certain instances where the player is fully lucid and has no headache, return to play is permissible. However, that player should be observed closely over the next 24 hours in case an expanding intracranial blood clot is developing. He should be awakened every 2 hours during the night and not be left alone that first night.

Whenever an injury involves a loss of consciousness, several important simultaneous observations and assumptions must be made. It must be assumed that the athlete has a fractured neck. The initial examination is crucial to subsequent evaluation and treatment. If the athlete shows improvement within a few minutes, subsequent transportation and diagnosis or evaluation can proceed in a routine manner. If, however, deterioration in the state of consciousness is seen, transportation and subsequent treatment must be expeditious. Every unconscious athlete should be transported on a fracture board. The head should be secured in a neutral position with sand bags, a four-poster collar, or a traction device if available.

If the unconscious athlete is wearing a helmet and has a good airway, the helmet should not be removed, since this may precipitate quadriplegia if an unstable cervical fracture is present. The helmet should be removed only if the airway is questionable, and then never forcibly and always with the neck in a neutral (neither flexed nor extended) position. The helmet can be used for cervical traction, with the chin strap serving as the halter and the earholes or the immediately adjacent edge of the helmet as a site for attaching neutral traction. While the unconscious athlete is being moved onto the spine board, the earholes of the helmet may also serve as a convenient site to insert one's index fingers to effect gentle neutral cervical traction. Only after appropriate cervical spine x-rays have ruled out a cervical spine fracture, malalignment, or instability can the helmet be safely removed from the unconscious athlete.

If a fracture board is not readily available to transport the unconscious athlete from the site of injury, a decision must be made either to wait for the ambulance to arrive with its stretcher or to move the athlete using the locked-arm technique. While I generally favor the former, it is true that if enough players or spectators are present, locking hands to elbows of individuals standing opposite each other provides a secure surface for moving an injured athlete a short distance. When transporting an unconscious athlete in this manner, one person applies neutral traction to the helmet or otherwise secures the head in a neutral position.

Occasionally head trauma will be sufficient to produce a degree of brain swelling (edema) over the ensuing 24 hours, which may result in a severe headache. Following a concussion, you should be free of headache at rest before resuming training, and free of headache at maximal exertion training before returning to competition.

The question of when the student or recreational athlete should return to competition after repeated concussions is still controversial. For the non-professional athlete, it is generally agreed that two concussions of grade II or III severity during any one season should exclude one from further participation that season. When the athlete is free of headache at maximal exertion and has a normal electroencephalogram (EEG), he may safely resume competition after a first concussion. However, before this is allowed, there should be a thorough review of the circumstances resulting in the concussion. If available, videotapes or game films should be reviewed by the player, the coach, and the trainer. It should be determined whether the player was using his head unwisely, illegally, or both. It will also reveal whether he was wearing the equipment correctly. Finally, the equipment itself should be checked to be certain it is worn properly and fits correctly.

Intracranial Hemorrhage (Blood Clot)

The leading cause of death from athletic head injury is intracranial hemorrhage, or blood clot. There are four types of hemorrhage, and since all four types may be fatal, rapid and accurate medical assessment as well as appropriate follow-up is mandatory.

An *epidural* or *extradural hematoma* is usually the most rapidly progressing intracranial hematoma. It is frequently associated with a fracture in the temporal bone, and results from a tear in one of the arteries supplying the covering (dura) of the brain. The hematoma accumulates inside the skull but outside the covering of the brain. It may progress quite rapidly and reach a fatal size in 30 to 60 minutes. There may sometimes but not always be a lucid interval; that is, the athlete may initially regain consciousness after the head trauma and then start to experience increasing headache and progressive deterioration in level of consciousness, as the clot accumulates and the intracranial pressure increases. This lesion, if present, will almost always be apparent within an hour or two after the time of injury. The brain substance is usually free from direct injury; thus, if the clot is promptly removed surgically, a full recovery is to be expected. Because this lesion is rapidly and universally fatal if missed, all athletes receiving a head injury should be very closely observed for the next

24 hours, preferably where full neurosurgical services are immediately available.

A *subdural hematoma* occurs between the brain surface and the dura (covering of the brain); that is, under the dura and directly on the brain. It often results from a torn vein running from the surface of the brain to the dura. It may also result from a torn venous sinus or even a small artery on the surface of the brain. With this injury, there is often associated injury to brain tissue. If a subdural hematoma requires surgery within the first 24 hours, mortality is high; this is not due to the clot itself, but to the associated brain damage. With a subdural hematoma that progresses rapidly, the athlete usually does not regain consciousness, and immediate neurosurgical evaluation is obviously necessary. Occasionally the brain itself will not be injured, and a subdural hematoma may develop slowly over a period of days or weeks. This chronic subdural hematoma, although often associated with headache, may initially be present with a variety of very mild, almost imperceptible mental, motor, or sensory signs and symptoms. Since its recognition and removal will lead to full recovery, it must always be suspected in an athlete who has previously sustained a head injury and who appears somewhat abnormal days or weeks later. A CAT scan of the head will definitively show such a lesion.

An *intracerebral hematoma* is the third type of intracranial hemorrhage seen after head trauma. In this instance, the bleeding is into the brain substance itself, usually from a torn artery. It may also result from the rupture of a congenital vascular lesion such as an aneurysm or an arteriovenous malformation. Intracerebral hematomas are not usually associated with a lucid interval and may be rapidly progressive. Death occasionally occurs before the injured athlete can be moved to a hospital. Because of the intense reaction such a tragic event precipitates among fellow athletes, family, students, and even the community at large, and the inevitable rumors that follow, it is imperative to obtain a complete autopsy to fully clarify the causative factors. Often the autopsy will reveal a congenital lesion, indicating that the cause of death was other than what had been presumed and was ultimately unavoidable. Only by such full, factual elucidation will inappropriate feelings of guilt in fellow athletes, friends, and family be assuaged.

The fourth type of intracranial hemorrhage is *subarachnoid,* or confined to the surface of the brain. Following head trauma, such bleeding results from disruption of the tiny surface brain vessels and is analogous to a bruise. As in intracerebral hematoma, there is often brain swelling, and such a hemorrhage can also result from a ruptured cerebral aneurysm or an arteriovenous malformation. Bleeding is superficial, and surgery is not usually required unless a congenital vascular anomaly is present.

All types of intracranial hemorrhages usually cause headache and, not infrequently, associated neurologic deficit, depending on the area of the brain involved. The irritative properties of the blood may also precipitate a seizure. If a seizure occurs in a head-injured athlete, it is important to log-roll the patient onto his or her side so that any blood or saliva will roll out of the mouth or nose and the tongue cannot fall back, obstructing the airway. A padded tongue depressor or oral airway can be inserted between the teeth. Under no circumstances should fingers be inserted into a seizing person's mouth, as a traumatic amputation can easily result from such an unwise maneuver. Traumatic seizure will usually last only for a minute or two; the athlete will then relax and can be transported to the nearest medical facility.

Skull Fractures

There are three basic types of skull fracture. The first is a linear fracture, which is best likened to a crack in the skull bone. The second is a depressed fracture, in which a portion of the bone is driven inward and may have to be surgically elevated. The third is a comminuted fracture, in which there are multiple fractures. If any of these three types of fractures have a laceration of the scalp overlying it, we use the term *compound* in front of the type, as in compound linear skull fracture. A compound fracture introduces the high risk of infection. Fractures, except with gross cranial disruption, are diagnosed by skull x-rays. They represent an indication of the force of head trauma, but unless depressed do not necessarily imply brain injury. Because of the risk of a possibly developing intracranial hematoma, anyone with a skull fracture should be under medical observation for at least 24 to 48 hours.

Sports Most Hazardous to the Head

Ranking at the top of the list of athletic pursuits most likely to cause head injury are automobile and motorcycle racing and hang gliding. Amazingly, adequate helmets are not even uniformly worn in this latter "sport." Football is the only team sport included in this most hazardous group. Thanks to the improved design of football helmets, especially the air helmet, serious football-related head injuries are now rare. While concussions are still fairly common, the incidence of intracranial hematoma is now very rare. (I will have more to say about football neck injuries in the next chapter.)

At this point, I wish to make a few comments about boxing, an activity I choose not to call a "sport." This is the only pursuit in which the intent is to hurt the opponent, and the head is the primary target. I have no aversion to professional boxing, which I personally enjoy watching. I regard this, however, as all other professional athletics, not as a sport but as entertainment. Whether it be Evil Kneivel attempting to jump a canyon on a motorcycle or Marvelous Marvin Hagler defending his middleweight boxing championship, these are paid professional entertainers taking known risks for monetary profit. I do not regard amateur boxing in the same light, because I do not believe most of the participants fully understand the potential risks of brain injury. How pathetic were the final two fights of Mohammed Ali. This great heavyweight champion, who once possessed perhaps the fastest hand-eye coordination of any heavyweight boxer, was now unable to unload even the simplest of boxing combinations. No, this was not due to his age, it was due to the many blows he had taken to the head. We know that in our late thirties and forever after, our endurance capacity slowly deteriorates. Next to go will be our speed and finally much, much later, will be our coordination. The fact that concert musicians remain active in their advanced senior years and the United States Tennis Association ranks tennis players into their eighties attests to just how long we can retain our coordination. No, don't feel sorry for Ali's present state of coordination. He made many tens of millions of dollars and placed himself in the record books. It is the young, nonprofessional boxer with much less talent, making no income and jeopardizing his future, that I am concerned about. For these reasons, I refuse to acknowledge amateur boxing as a sport, and, thus, you will not see it in any of the tables.

Prevention of Head Injuries

Prevention of athletic head injuries is largely limited to using appropriate protective headgear, such as the NOCSAE football helmet, and then taking one's chances. The brain cannot be preconditioned to accept trauma. Rather, the reverse is true: Once the brain is injured, it is more susceptible to future injury.

Eye Injuries

As with the head, for the eye, too, prevention is the key. Appropriate protective devices will eliminate most eye injuries, but even with the best protection and with enforcement of rules, injuries will still occur. This makes it especially important to consider the athlete with reduced vision in one eye. If one eye is normal, and the other has subnormal vision that cannot be corrected with glasses or contact lenses, the decision to participate in athletics rests on the quality of vision in the poor eye, and the chances of leading a normal life with the vision in the poor eye if a catastrophic injury occurred to the good eye. Best correctable vision of 20/40 or better is consistent with most normal activities. Best correctable vision between 20/50 and 20/200 makes it impossible to drive a car in most states and makes many jobs that require good vision impossible; yet, the person may still lead a productive life with the remaining vision. Best correctable vision below 20/200 is considered legally blind in most states and qualifies the patient for the benefits given the blind by society. An athlete should be considered one-eyed if the best corrected vision in the involved eye is 20/200 or less, with the other eye found normal by an ophthalmologist. Since the loss of the good eye would result in legal or total blindness, the athlete and the parents must be informed of the potential long-term consequences if the good eye is lost. They should also be informed of the risks of injury, the effectiveness of available protective devices, and the possibilities of repair of injuries typically seen with the sport in question. Boxing should be totally excluded from consideration, since there is no possibility of protecting the remaining eye. Collision and contact sports should be discouraged, since even with the best protectors, catastrophic eye injuries are possible. However, if the player, parents, and their lawyers (one cannot discriminate against the handicapped) are persistent after an informative discussion, they should sign appropriate waivers provided by the school committee legal staff. No waiver should be given for boxing; the protection of the athlete is worth a court appeal. The waiver should include mandatory use of protective devices. Class I or Class II sports eye protectors must be worn at all times while participating in *any* sport. In addition, appropriate helmet or face-mask protection is to be used for all practices and games.

In general, any person considered one-eyed should wear safety glasses most of the time to protect the good eye. This is especially true of young active people who are subject to injury on or off the athletic field.

Eye, face, and head protectors should be chosen and properly fitted to each athlete. Well-made, properly fitted protective devices are as important to the freshman team as they are to the varsity. If used equipment is recycled to less-skilled players, it should be of first quality and fit well. There is no place for obsolescent protective equipment in any athletic program.

If the athlete wears glasses, the type of lens and frame should be specified by the optician. Streetwear glasses may be unsafe for many sports, and a Class II eye protector should be required before athletic participation. If an athlete wears contact lenses, a back-up pair of eyeglasses should be required at all games and practices. Since contact lenses offer no eye protection, an appropriate eye protector must be worn for those sports where protection is necessary.

Athletes should be instructed on the importance of proper use and maintenance of protective gear. Failure to use the protective devices should result in a strict penalty, such as benching for the remainder of the practice or game.

The general principle for physicians treating all significant eye injuries is *patch and refer,* as more harm than good will result from improper attempts at treatment on the athletic field. With this in mind, as well as the ever-present danger of retinal detachment leading to blindness, almost all eye injuries (and at a later date all blunt trauma to the eye or orbit) should have an ophthalmological examination to rule out external and internal eye injury.

Eye Protection

Total-Head Protection Concept
Several sports (football, hockey, lacrosse) have such high-potential energy levels that the head, brain, face, eyes, teeth, jaw, and, in some

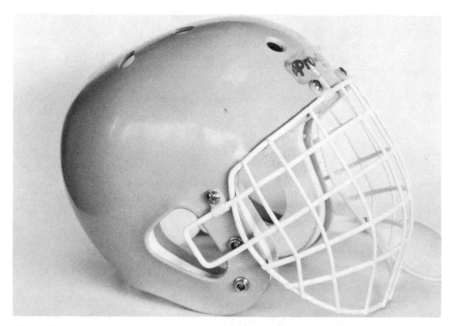

Figure 11–1. The helmet protects the brain, face, eyes, teeth and jaw from injury.

cases, the larynx must be protected as a unit. Forces are transmitted through a helmet-mounted face protector to a helmet designed to protect the brain (Figure 11-1).

Full-Face Protector

Some sports (fencing) have the potential for injury to the entire facial structure, but the forces are directed mostly from the front, with little threat to the brain. Energy is transmitted to the buttress bones of the face (frontal, zygoma, and maxilla) and the mandible (lower jaw) by padding at the periphery of the protector.

Sports Eye Protector

This device is designed to protect the eyes only. Several design options are available:

Class I: A protector with the lens and frame frontpiece molded as one unit. Frame temples or other devices (such as straps) to affix to the lens/ frontpiece may be separate pieces (Figure 11-2).

Class II: A protector with a lens, either nonprescription or prescription, mounted in a frame that is manufactured as a separate unit (Figure 11-3).

Class III: A protector without a lens, designed for use by itself or over spectacles. This is no longer recommended, because a ball may deform and protrude through this device and strike the eye (Figure 11-4).

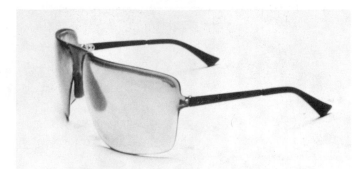

Figure 11–2. Protective glasses, class I. Reproduced with permission from *Sports Injuries, The Unthwarted Epidemic* edited by Paul F. Vinger and Earl F. Hoerner ©1981, Wright-PSG Publishing Co., Inc.

Larynx Protector

This device, worn separately or mounted onto a face protector, is designed to prevent blows to the larynx.

Mouth Injuries

Since the teeth have a lower potential for returning to a normal, healthy state than any other part of the body, and since attempts at reconstruction are costly and time consuming, the main emphasis should be on the choice of adequate protection. Full-face protectors (when indicated) should be chosen and well fitted to the helmet and face. For internal protection, a protector custom-made by a dentist is preferred over the stock-type and mouth-formed protectors. Most teams can enlist the assistance of a sports-minded dentist who will mold these guards for the entire team at lower cost as a service to the school. If the custom-made mouth guard is not within the team budget, the services of a dentist to aid in the forming of the kit-type mouth protectors will help assure proper fit and protection. Internal mouth protectors help reduce the incidence of tooth fracture, protect the jaw, and may help prevent concussion from blows to the chin. They should be made with a fail-safe strap to attach to the face guard for use in football and hockey to prevent possible aspiration of the protector.

Any dental prosthesis should be removed for contact sports, because there is the danger of the wearer being knocked unconscious aspirating the prosthesis.

The teeth and the stability and motion of the jaw should be examined after all blows to the mouth and chin. Athletes may resume play after a partially fractured (angle or corner) stable tooth where there is no pain or bleeding, but he or she should be seen by a dentist as soon as possible. Partially dislodged teeth require immediate dental evaluation for alignment and stabilization. Completely dislodged teeth should be repositioned into

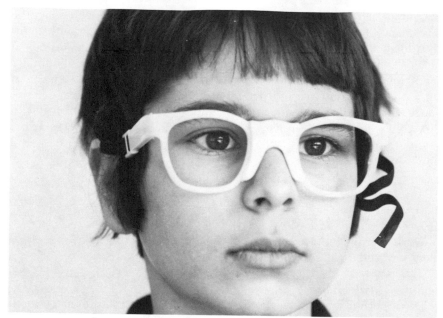

Figure 11–3. Protective glasses, class II. Reporduced with permission from *Sports Injuries, The Unthwarted Epidemic* edited by Paul F. Vinger and Earl F. Hoerner © 1981, Wright-PSG Publishing Co., Inc.

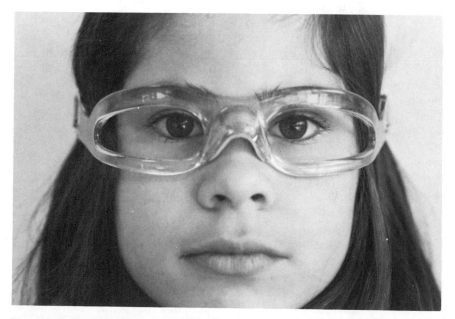

Figure 11–4. Protective glasses, class III. Reproduced with permission from *Sports Injuries, The Unthwarted Epidemic* edited by Paul F. Vinger and Earl F. Hoerner © 1981, Wright-PSG Publishing Co., Inc.

the gum if there appears to be no root fracture. If this cannot be done, the best chance of maintaining viability is to hold the tooth in your mouth under the tongue to keep it moist until it can be splinted by a dentist. A dislodged tooth should not be carried outside the mouth. If kept out of the mouth dry for 30 minutes, there is almost no chance of retention after replacement. If the athlete is unconscious or disoriented, the tooth should be carried in wet gauze. Bleeding in the mouth and surrounding tissue can be controlled with direct pressure while awaiting definitive care. A chest x-ray is necessary to rule out aspiration if missing teeth or a dental prosthesis cannot be found on the playing field.

Mouth Protection

External Mouth Guard
Worn over the mouth, this protector is designed to transmit forces away from the teeth to the maxilla (skull) and mandible (lower jaw).

Internal Mouth Guard
This device is worn between the teeth, to prevent fracture of the teeth and jaw. Several types are available: stock, mouth-formed, and custom-fabricated over a model.

Face Injuries

Since the facial skeleton is the supporting structure for the digestive tract, the most important consideration with any facial injury is the maintenance of an adequate airway. After a blow to the jaw or neck, a fractured larynx should be suspected if there is any change in the quality of the voice, shortness of breath, or hemorrhage. Fractures to the frontal bone, mid-face nose, zygoma (cheek bones), and jaw require a stabilization of the patient, maintenance of the airway, control of bleeding, and referral to a specialist's care.

Since the emphasis in this chapter has been almost totally on prevention, I wish to close with the following recommendations. First, total head protection (helmet, full-face protector, internal mouth guard) should be considered essential for football, hockey (forwards, defensemen, and goalies), lacrosse, box lacrosse, and baseball catchers, and is recommended for field hockey and baseball batters (especially Little League). Second, a helmet with separate eye protector is essential for auto racing, cycling, motorcycling, horseback riding, and snowmobiling and is suggested for polo and cricket. Third, a helmet alone is essential for boxing and a face protector for fencing. Finally, an eye protector is essential for racquet sports and is recommended for baseball, basketball, cross-country and downhill skiing, soccer, and softball.

Chapter 12

Spine Injuries

Cervical Spine Injuries

The same kinds of injuries that can happen to the brain—that is, concussion, contusion, and the various types of hemorrhage—may also occur to the cervical spinal cord. The major concern with a cervical spine injury is the possibility of an unstable fracture, which may produce quadriplegia. There is no way to determine the presence of an unstable fracture until appropriate x-rays are taken. Initially, there is also no way of differentiating a full recovery from a permanent case of quadriplegia. If one is fully conscious, the presence of a cervical fracture or cervical cord injury is usually accompanied by rigid cervical muscle spasm and pain, which immediately alerts one to the presence of such an injury. It is the unconscious athlete, who is unable to express pain and whose neck muscles are not in protective spasm, who is susceptible to potential cord severance if the possibility of an unstable cervical spine fracture is not considered. It is imperative that no neck manipulation be carried out on the field. Definitive treatment must await appropriate x-rays at a medical facility, and until such x-rays exclude the presence of a fracture, one must be assumed to be present.

In addition to neck injuries, a stretch or traction injury to the brachial plexus (nerves of the arm) or a nerve root must be considered. This condition, called a "burner," usually results from a forceful blow to the head from the side, but can also result from head extension or by depression of the shoulder while the head and neck are fixed. One experiences a shock-like sensation of pain and numbness radiating into the arm and hand. Repeated injury of this type over a period of years may lead to weakness of the deltoid, triceps, and teres major muscles (arm muscles), as well as constant pain. The use of a high cervical collar, which limits lateral neck

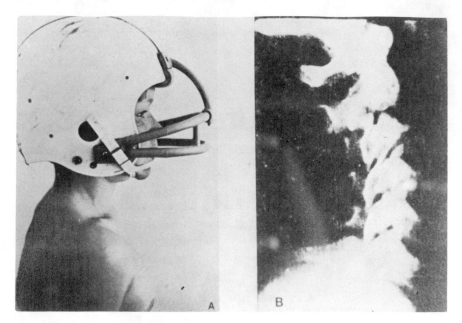

Figure 12–1. In neutral position the neck has a gently S-shaped curve. Reproduced with permission from *Sports Medicine in Primary Care* by Robert C. Cantu, M.D. © 1982 D.C. Heath and Company

flexion and extension, changing one's hitting technique, or moving to another position may eliminate this problem. If it recurs repeatedly, however, you should stop playing the responsible contact sport and move to another athletic pursuit.

If you sustain burner-like symptoms but the pain, numbness, and/or weakness persist (usually with neck pain and spasm), a ruptured cervical disc is to be suspected. Such a lesion often exists in a young athlete without any abnormality on routine cervical spine x-rays.

A final uncommon, but very serious, neck injury involves the carotid arteries (the arteries of the neck, face, and skull). The inner layer (intima) of the carotid may be torn by extremes of lateral flexion or extension or by a forceful blow from a relatively fixed narrow object, such as a stiffened forearm or a ski tip impaling one's neck in a forward fall. This can lead to a clot formation at the site of injury, resulting in emboli to the brain or, more commonly, a complete occlusion (blocking) of the artery, causing a major stroke.

It is recommended that an athlete not return to competition after a neck injury until he or she is free of any neck or arm pain at rest and has a full range of neck motion without discomfort or spasm. Further criteria used at Harvard University involve measuring the maximum weight each athlete can pull with neck in flexion, extension, and to each side. This becomes the neck profile for that athlete. An athlete with a neck injury is not allowed

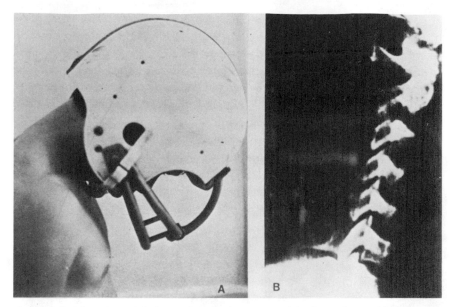

Figure 12–2. When the neck is flexed the spine becomes straight. Reproduced with permission from *Sports Medicine in Primary Care* by Robert C. Cantu, M.D. © 1982 D.C. Heath and Company.

to return to competition until he or she can perform at the level of his or her neck profile.

The most common mechanism of cervical spine injury in football is illustrated in Figures 12-1 and 12-2. In neutral posture, the neck has a gentle S-shaped curve (Figure 12-1). When the neck is flexed, the spine becomes straight (Figure 12-2). With the vertebral bodies lined up straight, vertical impact force is directly transmitted from one vertebra to the next, and little of the impact force can be absorbed by the muscles. If the impact force exceeds the strength of the bone, it compacts the bone at one or more levels, causing a compression fracture. If the fractured vertebra malaligns and is driven back into the spinal cord, quadriplegia may result.

It is when tackling with the head, especially in the open field where momentum is greatest, that most serious neck injuries occur. The small defensive back is the most susceptible player. The fast but light safety can be injured trying to bring down a larger, heavier back with a head tackle. The high-school athlete, who has the greatest degree of variation in physical maturation and athletic ability, is at greatest risk.

Presently, catastrophic football head and neck injuries are at the lowest level in the last 18 years, approximately 0.5 per 100,000 athletes. This represents a reduction of over 600% from peak years in the late 1960s and directly reflects the 1976 rule change to prohibit butt-blocking and face-tackling. It is also due to the football helmet standard established by the

137

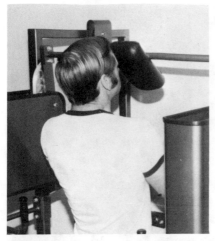

Figure 12–3

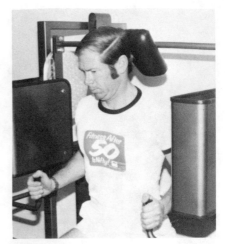

Figure 12–4

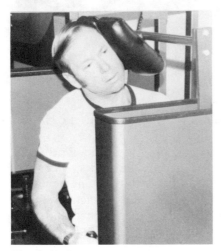

Figure 12–5

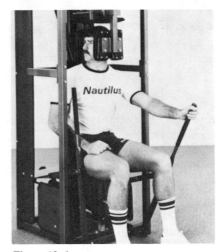

Figure 12–6

Figures 12–3 to 12–6 demonstrate how Nautilus machines can be used to strengthen neck muscles.

National Operating Committee on Standards for Athletic Equipment (NOCSAE), improved conditioning programs, and improved supervision by team physicians and trainers.

While football fatalities and catastrophic injuries will never be totally eliminated, their occurrence is now rare. Most football conferences go for decades without such an occurrence, while almost every participating school has one or more fatality or catastrophic injury attributed to a car or motorcycle accident each year. For the high school student, it is clearly more dangerous to drive a car or motorcycle than to play football.

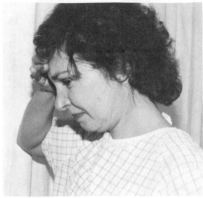

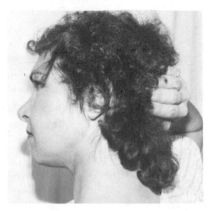

Figure 12–7   Figure 12–8

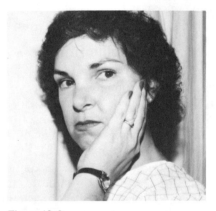

Figure 12–9

Figures 12–7 to 12–9 demonstrate neck strengthening exercises you can carry out with your own wrist.

Prevention of Neck Injuries

In contrast to the brain, the neck can be strengthened and the risk of injury reduced. Nautilus machines are now available that strengthen the neck in all four movements: flexion, extension, lateral bending, and rotation (Figs. 12-3 to 12-6). These same exercises can be carried out without machines using the resistance of your own or someone else's wrist (Figs. 12-7 to 12-9). While controversy exists as to whether the neck can be conditioned to withstand the maximum forces to which it may be subjected in contact sports, it is universally agreed that a neck exercise program minimizes the risk of neck injury.

Finally, since most serious neck injuries occur in diving accidents, and almost all occur in unsupervised recreation, the following tips should be kept in mind:

1. Never dive into unfamiliar water.

2. Do not assume the water is deep enough. Even familiar lakes, rivers, and swimming holes change levels.

3. If you are present when a spinal cord injury occurs, keep the victim's head and neck from bending and twisting.

4. Never dive near dredging or construction work. The water level may have dropped, and dangerous objects may be just beneath the surface.

5. Do not drink before diving or swimming. Alcohol distorts judgment.

6. Water around a raft can be dangerous, especially if the water level is down. A slackened cable permits the raft to drift, putting the cable and anchor into the diving area.

7. Cloudy water can conceal hazardous objects. Check the bottom.

Lumbar Spine Injuries

As a neurosurgeon, the most common medical problems I see are not brain tumors, ruptured cerebral aneurysms, strokes, or spinal cord injuries, but spine problems involving disorders of the lower back. For me, this is gratifying, because most brain tumors are malignant and incurable, while almost all spine problems are correctable.

At one time or another, almost everyone will experience low back pain. A recent U.S. Public Health Service report indicates that 7 million Americans have experienced at least one severe, incapacitating, prolonged episode of low back pain. Our National Center for Health Statistics states that chronic and recurring back ailments form the largest single medical ailment. Today, low back pain represents a major national health problem, with more than $15 billion being spent annually on the treatment and compensation of people who suffer from low back problems. In industry, compensation for low back problems represents a figure in excess of the cost of all other industrial injuries combined.

Experience in sports medicine indicates that low back problems are a very common ailment in the athlete and nonathlete alike. The medical team for the Canadian athletes at the 1976 Olympic Games found low back pain to be a common problem in their highly trained athletes. Many outstanding Olympic athletes tolerate low back pain as a constant problem, and in some cases the disorder has progressed to the point of neurologic involvement, even though the athlete is still competing.

What are the causes of low back pain? Why are young, vigorous, physically fit male and female athletes suffering from the same symptoms that are so prevalent in the unfit, sedentary middle-aged person? The cause of low back pain is usually mechanical, either a strain of the back muscles or improper postural alignment (with or without weakness of certain muscles). Fortunately, this problem can be successfully treated in most people with the simple back exercises, a postural correction program, and the helpful hints outlined in this chapter. There is a correct way to sit, walk, stand, and carry out normal activities of daily living so that the low back and pelvis are in the correct postural alignment. Likewise, there is a correct way to lift. Those with low back problems must learn to avoid certain movements and activities that place excessive stress in this area of the body.

A small percentage of people with low back problems will not only have low back pain, but also pain that radiates from the back into the buttock and/or down one or both legs. Coughing, sneezing, and straining to pass urine or a bowel movement usually makes the leg pain worse. There may be numbness, usually in the foot either over the medial half or along the lateral side. This pattern of pain is called *sciatica* and suggests that a ruptured disc is pressing on a nerve root.

Discs are the fibrocartilagenous cushions between the vertebrae. As we age, they lose fluid content, becoming slightly narrower, and cause all of us to shrink slightly in height. The outer, more fibrous capsule of the disc, called the *annulus fibrosus,* may also tear, allowing the disc to rupture in the back of the disc space and compress the nerve root as it exits from the spine. Most simple ruptures can be treated successfully with a period of bedrest, muscle relaxants, anti-inflammatory medicines, analgesics, and, later, exercises. A minor percentage of sufferers with neurological deficits (such as a reflex absence at knee or ankle, weakness of ankle or great toe extension, or persistent pain and numbness) will require surgical excision of the ruptured disc. The success of such surgery should exceed 90%. Following surgery, the patient should adhere to the exercises and advice given in this chapter.

A third and very small group of people with low back problems suffer from mechanical malalignment of the vertebrae, called *spondylolisthesis.* This diagnosis is established by an x-ray of the back. If there is instability, documented by further malalignment as the back is placed through flexion and extension maneuvers, then a surgical procedure of lumbar fusion may be indicated.

Another small group of people may experience back pain due to an abnormal lateral curvature of the spine called *scoliosis.* In children, severe scoliosis may require surgical correction, which is an extensive and time consuming procedure. For most, however, the scoliosis is mild and can be pain free if the exercises and hints in this chapter are followed. Only a physician, and especially an orthopedist or neurosurgeon, is properly qualified to evaluate and treat your low back problem. Therefore, the exercises and advice in this chapter are directed primarily at the person with low back pain but without neurologic deficit, or the person who has already had concern for a ruptured disc or spinal instability eliminated by appropriate medical consultation.

The Mechanism of Low-Back Strain

The lower back is composed of five mobile lumbar vertebrae with carti-lagenous cushions, or discs, between them, and the fused bones of the sacrum and coccyx, which form the back of the pelvis. It is in the area of the lumbar vertebrae that all forward (flexion) and backward (extension) movement of the back occurs. Movement is greatest, and, thus, stress is greatest, between the sacrum and fifth lumbar vertebrae and between the fourth and fifth lumbar vertebrae. That is why more than 80% of all lumbar disc ruptures occur at those levels. Because the lumbar spine curves for-ward, the vertebrae are supported by the back muscles, much in the same way as a leaning pole may be supported by guy wires.

The position of the pelvis, which is controlled by the hip and abdominal muscles, affects the position of the low back. The forward curvature of the low back increases when the upper pelvis rotates forward and downward. The result is a swayback appearance or what is medically termed increased *lumbar lordosis*. This position causes the muscles and ligaments of the back to become shortened and tight. Pain may result without exertion and almost certainly will appear with any sudden movement or motion. This condition occurs when there is weakness of the abdominal muscles and the gluteal muscles of the buttocks.

For most, however, it occurs when care is not taken to achieve good posture, the position of one's body during activity and rest. Good posture is achieved by rotating the top of the pelvis backward, which flattens the curve in the low back. The section on exercises in this chapter is designed to strengthen the abdominal and gluteal muscles and stretch out tight back muscles. When this is achieved, lordosis is replaced with a flat low back, and the symptoms of strain—namely pain—will vanish.

Almost all athletic injuries to the lower back involve either a contusion (a bruise from a direct blow), a sprain (a pulling with stretching and tearing of the muscles or their tendons), or a strain (tearing of a ligament). In general, a strain is most painful when the back is forced in the opposite direction, and a sprain produces pain when the affected muscle is con-tracted. There is an intricate relationship among the muscles, tendons, and ligaments of the back, and most injuries involve two or all three entities.

The cause of most back strains and sprains in athletes and nonathletes is weak muscles (especially the abdominal muscles and hip flexors) or lack of flexibility (especially in the hamstring hip extensor muscles). One wonders how world class athletes could have weak muscles. During intensive train-ing, world class athletes often neglect anatomic areas (the back, abdomen, or hip) that do not seem to require development for success in their sport. At the 1976 Olympics, the Canadian medical team found the abdominal muscles underdeveloped in many world class athletes. Some of Canada's top athletes had trouble executing more than one or two bent-knee sit-ups.

142

In general, athletes have strong extensor muscles (the back and hip), and the flexor muscles in one or both regions are frequently underdeveloped.

Most strains and sprains develop in one of two ways. The first is by a sudden, abrupt, violent extension/contraction of an overloaded, unprepared, or underdeveloped spine, especially when there is some rotation in the attempted movement. This can result in stretching a few fibers, a complete tear, or an avulsion fracture of a vertebrae spinous or transverse process. The second mechanism involves a chronic strain, often with associated poor posture and excessive lumbar lordosis. There is a continuation of the underlying disease with recurring injury to the original and adjacent sites.

Through the repetition of training, many sports predispose to low back pain. Most sports involve either strong back-extension movements, as opposed to strong flexion, or external forces that produce extension. Track athletes run in forced extension. The discus thrower, shot putter, and weight lifter propel heavy weights with the back extended. Gymnasts repeatedly dismount with a hyperextended low back as the feet hit the mat. The diver hits the water in extension with foot-entry dives.

Treatment

The successful treatment of low back pain in athletes involves a three-step program: (1) relief of pain and spasm; (2) adoption of an appropriate exercise program that includes both stretching and strengthening exercises; and (3) an educational program that considers the training program and is tailored to prevent future injuries.

Relief of Pain and Spasm

Ice, analgesics, muscle relaxants, anti-inflammatory agents, and rest are used in acute stages. Heat, muscle stimulation, ultrasound, physical therapy, and the same pharmacologic agents are used 12 or more hours after injury. Ultrasound and gentle muscle stimulation seem to dissipate muscle spasm, and relieve tenderness and general soreness more rapidly. This is probably due to enhanced muscle circulation and exchange at the cellular level of prescribed pharmacologic agents, plus elimination of toxic cellular products. Actually, while modes of pain relief exist, no one treatment has been clearly demonstrated to accelerate actual tissue healing.

Stretching and Strengthening Exercises

Medication, manipulation, massage, ultrasound, and hot and cold applications do not strengthen a weakened or compromised part of the body. Low back pain is usually due to muscles that are weak, tense, fatigued, or all three. Once the healing process has occurred, it is essential to begin an exercise program to rebuild the back and abdominal musculature.

The 10 basic low back exercises that are listed in Table 12-1 and illustrated in Chapter 4 constitute a potent, effective means of eliminating low

143

Table 12-1

Exercise Title	Exercise Number
Back Flattener	6
Single Knee Raise	13
Single Knee Hug	14
Double Knee Hug	15
Single Leg Raise	16
Partial Sit-up	24
Advanced Sit-up	25
Advanced Mod. Sit-up	26
Sitting Bend	27
Deep Knee Bend	29
Posture Check	8

back pain. They can easily be done in less than 15 minutes per day and should be performed daily for maximum effectiveness. Unless specifically prescribed by a physician, these exercises should *not* be done by a person with sciatica (pain radiating from the back, out and down the leg). Sciatica involves irritation of one or more nerve roots as they leave the spine. It is usually due to traction or stretching of a nerve root, or pressure on a root from a ruptured disc. Sciatica may be aggravated by these exercises.

Even in the absence of sciatica, the exercises should not be done if severe back pain is experienced at rest. Wait until the back pain is gone before embarking on the exercise program.

The exercises should be carried out on a hard, flat surface with adequate padding. A tumbling mat is ideal, but a thick rug with underpadding is fine. A thick blanket or quilt added to a thin rug will also suffice. A pillow placed under your neck for those exercises done lying down will make you more comfortable. Wear loose clothing or underclothes.

One must be cautious not to overdo in the beginning. The exercises must always be started slowly and carefully to allow muscles to loosen up gradually. Never use jerking or snapping movements. Relaxing before exercising aids in achieving the maximum benefit from the exercises. Heat treatments before you start can help tight muscles. Do not be alarmed if the exercises produce some mild-to-moderate discomfort, which may persist for up to a half-hour. If frank pain occurs and does not vanish quickly with cessation of the exercises, do no more exercises until you have checked with your doctor, preferably a neurosurgeon or orthopedist.

The exercises should be done every day, twice a day in the beginning. If you are unable to exercise most days of the week, it is better not to do them at all than to exercise once or twice a week. Many people find it most convenient to do them when they first get up in the morning and again at

144

night just before retiring. Others, bored by the exercises, find that doing them while the TV set is on relieves the monotony.

Each person should progress at his or her own pace. Three repetitions of every exercise for the first 7 days is recommended. Then, one may add a repetition or two daily to each exercise, repetitions that can be done with relative ease and comfort. In this way, gradually build to the minimum desired number of repetitions as later outlined for each exercise.

It cannot be stressed too strongly that all exercises must be executed slowly and smoothly. If one or more of the exercises produces significant discomfort, it should be discontinued for several days while the remainder are carried out. An attempt to resume the exercise very slowly, smoothly, and carefully, with fewer repetitions, can then be made several days later. If pain is experienced even then, do not resume that exercise without first checking with your doctor.

Educational Program

The final step in eliminating low back pain involves educating the athlete to avoid back problems, both in training and in daily life. common everyday tips to avoid the occurrence of low back pain include the following:

Sitting:

1. Sit so that your lower back is flat or slightly rounded outward, never with a forward curve.

2. Sit so that your knees are higher than your hips; this may require a small footstool.

3. Hard chair backs that begin contact with your back four to six inches above the seat, and provide a flat support throughout the entire lumbar area, are preferable.

4. Do not sit on soft or overstuffed chairs or sofas.

5. Avoid sitting in swivel chairs or chairs on rollers.

6. Never sit in the same position for prolonged periods; get up and move around.

Driving:

1. Push the front seat forward so that your knees will be higher than your hips, and the pedals are easily reached without stretching.

2. Sit with your back flat; do not lean forward.

3. Add a flat back-rest if your seat is soft or if you are traveling a long distance.

4. If on a long trip, stop every 30 to 60 minutes, get out of your car, and walk for several minutes, tensing buttocks and abdomen to flatten back.

5. Always fasten seat belt and shoulder harness.

6. Be sure your car seat has a properly adjusted headrest.

Bed Rest:

1. Sleep or rest only on a flat, firm mattress. If one is not available, place a bedboard of not less than ¾-inch plywood under the mattress. A board of less thickness will sag, preventing proper spine alignment.

2. When sleeping, the preferred position is on your side, both arms in front, and knees slightly drawn up toward your chin.

3. When lying on your back, place a pillow under your knees, because raising the legs flattens the lumbar curve.

4. When lying in bed, do not extend your arms above your head; relax them at your side.

5. If your doctor prescribes absolute bed rest, stay in bed. Raising your body or twisting and turning can strain your back.

Lifting:

1. When lifting, let the legs do the work, using the large muscles of the thighs instead of the small muscles of the back.

2. Squat directly in front of the object you plan to lift, bending your knees and going down as far as necessary with the legs, not the back.

3. Do not twist your body; face the object.

4. Never lift with your legs straight.

5. Do not lift heavy objects from car trunks.

6. Do not lift from a bending-forward position.

7. Do not reach over furniture to open and close windows.

8. Tuck in the buttocks and pull in the abdomen when lifting.

9. Lift holding the object close to your body.

10. Lift a heavy load no higher than your waist, a light load no higher than the shoulders, as greater height increases lumbar lordosis.

11. To turn while lifting, pivot your feet, turning your whole body at one time.

Standing and Walking:

1. Stand with your low back erect and as flat as possible.

2. Bend at the knees when you must lean, as when leaning over a wash basin. Avoid leaning whenever possible, and squat with a straight lower back if possible.

3. Avoid high-heeled shoes; they shorten your Achilles tendons and increase lumbar lordosis.

4. Avoid standing for long periods of time, but if you must, alternate left foot and right foot, and if possible use the bent-knee position (as on a stool).

5. When standing, do not lean back and support your back with your hands. Keep your hands in front of your body and lean forward slightly.

6. When turning to walk from a standing position, move your feet first, and they your body.

7. Open doors widely enough to walk through comfortably.

8. Carefully judge the height of curbs before stepping up or down.

In training, to minimize back injuries, the athlete should always warm up slowly and cool down after the main workout. Both the warm-up and cooling-off periods should include back-stretching exercises. Calisthenics that involve hyperextension of the back, such as back bends, straight leg sit-ups, or straight leg raises, should be avoided when possible. By faithfully carrying out a daily program of back exercises, the athlete can pursue a variety of potentially hazardous sports with minimal risk of back injury.

Sports Most Hazardous to the Back

Table 12-2 lists some popular sports and the risk of injury they entail. Football is felt by some to be legalized assault, often between physical unequals. It is one of the most hazardous sports to the body, particularly

Table 12-2

	Injury To	
	Neck	**Low Back**
Archery	L	L
Automobile racing	H	M
Baseball	L	M
Basketball	L	M
Bicycling	L	L
Bowling	L	M
Diving	M	M
Football	H	H
Golf	L	L
Gymnastics	M	H
Handball	M	M
Hang gliding	H	H
Ice hockey	M	M
Ice-skating	L	L
Lacrosse	H	H
Motorcycle racing	H	H
Racquetball	M	M
Roller-skating	L	L
Rowing	L	M
Rugby	H	H
Running	L	L
Skiing	M	M
Soccer	M	M
Squash	M	M
Swimming	L	L
Tennis	M	M
Volleyball	M	M
Water skiing	M	M
Weight lifting	M	H
Wrestling		

L = low risk of injury   M = moderate risk of injury   H = high risk of injury to the back. This is especially true for the interior linemen (defensive ends, guards, tackles, and centers). A report from a major university with a high national ranking stated that during one year, 50% of its interior linemen sought medical attention for low back pain. This report postulated the biomechanics of back injury. As the lineman drives forward, attempting to push the opponent backward, the lumbar spine is extended; this converts more of the force to a shearing force that can lead to pars interarticularis injury. The report concluded that the high incidence of spondylolisthesis (displaced vertebrae) and spondylosis (broken down vertebrae) seen in interior linemen is the result of repeated forces being transmitted to the pars interarticularis while players are in the lumbar-extended posture.

Weight lifting, especially the overhead military press and the clean and jerk, is another high-risk back injury sport. Severe lordotic postures (when the back is concave) are also assumed when spiking a volleyball, hitting a twist serve or deep overhead stroke in tennis, putting the shot, throwing the discus or hammer, or even stretching for the tape in track. Extreme backward arching movements are required by the gymnast (especially in dismounts), diver, and trampolinist, and those who play squash, soccer, handball, and racquetball. Sledding, downhill skiing, and snow- and water-ski jumping can also result in excessive stress to the lower back. Both the hang-glider and pole-vaulter occasionally have precipitous descents in awkward postures that can result in back strain and even compression fractures.

Sports that are less likely to result in back injury include baseball, basketball, bowling, golf, figure skating, softball, ping-pong, waterskiing, canoeing, rowing, fencing, cross-country skiing, badminton, and archery. Sports least likely to result in back injuries include bicycling, hiking, swimming, fishing, curling, darts, skindiving, boccie, billiards, pool, and sailing.

In some sports, the most hazardous maneuvers can be modified. For example, the serve and the overhead are the two tennis strokes most strenuous to the back. By tossing a serve slightly forward, less back extension is required, causing less back strain. For those who play a serve and volley game, it will also aid in gaining forward momentum toward the net. When hitting the overhead, the player should go up to the ball, hitting it slightly in front of the body. When trying for a low ball, as in tennis, handball, volleyball, softball, or baseball, the athlete should bend the knees rather than the back, whenever possible. Most gymnastic sports and diving stress good posture. The athlete should sit and stand as tall as possible at all times. The runner, equestrian, diver, and gymnast should keep the lower back flat by tensing the buttocks and abdominal muscles whenever possible.

Chapter 13

Chest, Abdomen, and Genitourinary Tract Injuries

Injuries to the chest, abdomen, and genitourinary system can occur wtih any activity that involves rapid deceleration or impact to these regions. Collision sports such as football, lacrosse, or hockey are especially likely to produce torso injuries. The most common thoracic (chest) and abdominal injuries include contusion (bruise), abrasion, fracture, muscle strain, ligament sprain, and laceration. If the injury is superficial, recognition is usually obvious; but intense injuries are often very difficult to diagnose, requiring medical evaluation, often by a specialist. Table 13-1 lists the injury risks to the chest, abdomen, and genitourinary tract by sport.

It is especially helpful with chest injuries if you and your fellow athletes know cardiopulmonary resuscitation (CPR). CPR courses are offered free or at a nominal cost by most community hospitals as well as the Red Cross. It truly can make the difference between life and death.

Although it happened several years ago, the pain of remembering the loss of a friend and fellow racket sport player still lingers. At the time of his death, he was 44 years old and had just completed three vigorous sets of paddle tennis. Returning home that fall Sunday morning, Bret (not his real name) decided to go out for a brief jog, a pursuit he did not regularly pursue. He was stricken with a heart attack (cardiac arrhythmia) while jogging and fell to the roadside. Two individuals, tragically uninformed about CPR, came upon Bret. Both left Bret, one to call his wife and the other to call the police. When the police arrived some 10 minutes later, Bret was quite dead. His heart at autopsy showed a moderate cardiomyopathy (as discussed in Chapter 9). If those two people who came upon Bret had

Table 13-1
Injury To

	Chest	Abdomen	Genitourinary Tract
Archery	L	L	L
Automobile racing	H	H	H
Baseball	M	M	M
Basketball	M	M	M
Bicycling	L	L	L
Bowling	L	L	L
Diving	L	L	L
Football	H	H	H
Golf	L	L	L
Gymnastics	L	M	L
Handball	L	L	L
Hang gliding	H	H	H
Ice hockey	M	M	M
Ice-skating	L	L	L
Lacrosse	H	H	H
Motorcycle racing	H	H	H
Racquetball	M	M	M
Roller-skating	L	L	L
Rowing	L	L	L
Rugby	H	H	H
Running	L	L	M
Skiing	L	L	L
Soccer	L	L	L
Squash	M	M	M
Swimming	L	L	L
Tennis	L	L	L
Volleyball	L	L	L
Water skiing	M	M	L
Weight lifting	L	L	L
Wrestling	M	M	M

L = low risk of injury   M = moderate risk of injury   H = high risk of injury

known CPR, almost certainly he would be alive today. How reassuring it is to know that my son has already had a CPR course during his sophomore year of high school. All of us, especially recreational athletes, should be trained in CPR.

Chest Injuries

As is true for any major injury, the first priority with a chest injury is to make certain there is an adequate airway and that the athlete is breathing well. It must be quickly established that the victim is not obstructing the airway with his tongue, aspirated gum, a mouth guard, or other foreign body. It must be rapidly determined if he or she can breathe deeply and has full chest-wall excursion (range of movement). The presence or absence of a penetrating chest injury or flail segment of ribs with paradoxical motion in breathing (i.e., retraction of a segment while the remainder of the rib cage expands, and vice versa) must be determined. A quick assessment of circulation must also be part of the initial examination. This assessment should be orderly, thoughtful, thorough, and rapid, taking 30 to 60 seconds.

Players with puncture or penetrating wounds should be transported to a hospital immediately. Superficial abrasions should be cleansed with a sterile soap and covered with an occlusive sterile bandage. Lacerations (cuts) should be similarly cleansed and bandaged, and then medical attention should be sought.

Severe blunt injuries to the chest or abdomen require that the athlete be removed from the playing field and undergo medical examination for external injuries. Ice should be applied to the site of trauma to minimize tissue bleeding and hematoma (clot) formation. If pain increases, or pallor, sweating, and rapid pulse develop, the injured player should be speedily transferred to the hospital for general or thoracic surgical evaluation. The components of the chest wall, musculotendinous attachments, bone, soft tissue, and ligaments interact. The function of the upper extremities is also intimately associated with the thorax. Because the manubrium, sternum, and xiphoid (together, the breastbone) are covered by only skin and scant connective tissue, they are especially vulnerable to blunt trauma such as contusion with hematoma formation.

Contusion (bruise) of the sternum is best treated with ice and anti-inflammatory agents (such as aspirin) for the first 24 hours. Then heat (wet or dry) may replace the ice while the anti-inflammatory agents are continued. Activity should be limited until a full range of motion of the upper extremities and thorax is possible without pain. If a contact sport is being played, protective padding or even a fiberglass sheild is recommended with resumption of contact. Fractures of the sternum are fortunately uncommon, but if sternal pain does not subside in several days, x-rays are recommended.

Costochondral or costosternal subluxation or dislocation—partial or complete dislocation of the ribs or sternum—occur with deformity of the rib at its insertion. When present, evaluation by a thoracic surgeon is suggested. While it is easy to reduce manually—that is, to restore the parts to their proper positions—reduction is usually difficult to maintain. Costovertebral subluxation (partial dislocation of ribs and vertebrae) is painful and disabling and occasionally requires open reduction or resection. The initial treatment is ice, anti-inflammatory pain medication, and use of a rib belt. The athlete should not return to play until pain and tenderness are gone,

151

usually in 2 to 4 weeks. If pain persists longer than a month, referral to a thoracic surgeon is recommended.

Breast injuries are occurring with increasing frequency. This is because more women are participating in sports, and because of the current fad of not wearing bras. Wearing a firm-fitting bra will protect the breast from blunt trauma and from motion, which strains the fascial attachments of the breast to the pectoralis major muscle, resulting in pain. Breast contusions are treated like contusions elsewhere—that is, with immediate ice and anti-inflammatory pain medication followed later by heat and padding.

Gynecomastia (breast enlargement) may occur in young men. Frequently unilateral, the nipple may become sore, tender to pressure, and irritated from rubbing against the shirt. Female long-distance runners who do not wear bras may also suffer from nipple chafing. Wearing a proper bra may prevent this problem in women, and men may obtain relief by placing either vaseline or a single layer of plastic tape over their nipples. Gynecomastia is usually a self-limiting problem. If it persists, you should see an endocrinologist.

Rib fractures necessitate removal from competition, and the athlete should return only when (1) rib x-rays show healing of the fracture, (2) tenderness to palpation and compression is minimal, (3) no analgesic agent is required, and (4) full range of motion is possible. The early treatment is an analgesic agent for pain; while taping is no longer recommended, a canvas rib belt with shoulder straps may afford substantial relief, especially for sleeping. It is removed for bathing. Upon return to competition in collision sports, a flak jacket or fiberglass protective support is useful. "Cutter Cast" material is especially useful for this purpose.

The *musculotendinous attachments* to the thorax (pectoralis, latissimus dorsi, trapezius, rhomboid, and rectus muscles) may be strained by vigorous muscular contraction. Treatment, as for strains elsewhere, consists of initial application of ice plus oral anti-inflammatory, analgesic medication and decreased motion through the use of a sling. Rehabilitation can include heat, ultrasound, muscle-resistant exercises, and gradual resumption of activity. Cardiovascular fitness can be maintained during this period by bicycling or jogging.

Prevention of Chest Injuries

There is no absolute way to condition against chest injuries other than wearing appropriate protective equipment, depending on the sport. Chest injuries usually occur when excesses of trauma are absorbed largely by the skeletal system, as opposed to muscles. While it is certainly helpful to have well-developed pectoral, latissimus dorsi, and shoulder muscles (see Chapter 14, Figs. 14-7 to 14-11), their development cannot prevent chest wall or internal injuries. Thus, as is true for the head, eye, face, and mouth, so, too, with the chest, prevention primarily by appropriate protection is the key.

152

Abdominal Injuries

The abdominal wall is usually not the site of serious injury. This is because the abdomen is largely protected; it is on the flexion side of the torso and is soft compared to joints and the back, affording some give when it is struck. Also, players such as goalies, catchers, and fencers, who are the targets of thrown or propelled objects, usually wear well-designed and well-fitted protective padding. Injuries to the abdominal wall may be defined in several ways: (1) level of injury (skin, subcutaneous tissue, muscles); (2) blunt or penetrating; and (3) individually contracted (strains) or the result of contact with another athlete or an immovable object. All penetrating injuries should be seen by a general surgeon. Injuries individually contracted tend to be less severe than those resulting from a collision.

Injuries to the *skin* are minor, with abrasions resulting from friction burns being the most common. Through cleansing to eliminate surface dirt and debris is mandatory; then the wound should be covered with a light, occlusive, nonadhering dressing. Lacerations of the abdominal wall are uncommon, and their treatment is the same as for lacerations elsewhere. A note of caution is that abdominal subcutaneous fat is less resistant to infection than subcutaneous tissue elsewhere. Thus, there must be meticulous cleansing and removal of foreign debris. If the skin is penetrated, a tetanus immunization is suggested. If there is any question that the laceration extends into the abdominal wall muscle, general surgical consultation is advised.

The only injury of note at the subcutaneous level is a hematoma—arteriolar or venous bleeding into the fatty layer resulting from blunt trauma. Initial treatment should be ice for the first 24 to 48 hours, then heat. If recurrent hematomas develop in a young athlete, he or she should be screened for an underlying blood disorder such as leukemia or idiopathic thrombocytopenic purpura. It is recommended that all young athletes involved in contact sports have a complete blood count and urinalysis as part of their routine preseason physical examination.

The *muscles* of the *abdominal wall* protect the intra-abdominal viscera from most injury, but are themselves the site of very painful and debilitating injury. They include the two rectus muscles running parallel from the costal margins to the pelvis, the external and internal oblique muscles, and the transversus abdominis muscle lying closest to the peritoneal membrane. Injuries to the abdominal muscles can be grouped into blunt trauma (contusion), strain, and penetrating injuries. All penetrating injuries should be referred to a general surgeon. A rupture of the deep epigastric arteris and/or veins, creating a deep hematoma (clot) in the rectus-muscle sheath until self-tamponading occurs (that is, until enough pressure can be exerted to stop a hemorrhage), is the most serious blunt trauma injury of the abdominal wall. If the hematoma continues to enlarge, surgical referral is required, because removal of the hematoma and tying off the epigastric vessel is occasionally required. Treatment of this and lesser contusions of the abdominal wall include ice and anti-inflammatory/analgesic medication initially, then heat. When tenderness has abated and ability to perform all essential maneuvers has returned, the athlete is ready to return to competition. Obviously, no athlete on anti-coagulant medication should be allowed to participate in sports where blunt abdominal trauma may occur.

Abdominal muscle strains usually occur from overstretching a bundle of muscle fibers beyond their normal tensile capability, often when the torso is twisted and hyperextended in contact with another athlete or immovable object. The rectus muscle is essential for a wide variety of movements by hurdlers, ice skaters, rowers, and wrestlers, and is especially prone to strain. Strains can also occur when musculotendinous insertions are pulled away from the bone, such as the iliac crest (hip pointer), or when muscle fibers are pulled away from aponeurotic sheaths or lines. With a hip pointer in a young athlete before growth plate closure, the bone may be avulsed (or torn off). An x-ray to rule out fracture or epiphyseal separation is required. The iliopsoas muscle is prone to strain in divers and gymnasts. Rupture that requires removal of a retroperitoneal hematoma and control of bleeding points rarely occurs.

The treatment of muscle strains here is the same as elsewhere: ice to minimize secondary tissue damage from bleeding, and pain and anti-inflammatory medication; after 48 hours, local heat should be applied to improve arteriolar blood supply necessary for normal healing.

Internal Abdominal Injuries

Internal abdominal injuries are less common than abdominal wall injuries. However, failure to promptly recognize such injuries can lead to severe morbidity and loss of life. Early abdominal signs of viscera injury are often subtle. With this in mind, when intra-abdominal injury with blunt trauma is suspected, and in all cases of penetrating abdominal injury, referral to a general surgeon or traumatologist is recommended.

After blunt abdominal trauma, the most reliable physical finding indicating peritoneal irritation is the presence of voluntary or involuntary spasm, or both. Spasm can best be detected by gently placing the palm of the hand on the abdominal muscle over the rectus muscle, having the patient breathe deeply, and gently depressing the examining hand with the other hand. As the patient exhales, voluntary spasm of the rectus muscle will abate, involuntary spasm will not, and the muscle will feel tense and boardlike. The exact area of tenderness should be localized with one finger and will give a clue as to the viscus injured. In addition, when the hand pressing the tender area is quickly removed, rebound tenderness may be felt in the primary site of pain. This provides further evidence of peritoneal irritation. If any signs of peritoneal irritation, or voluntary or involuntery

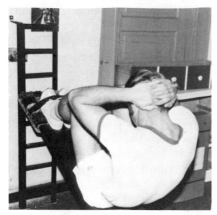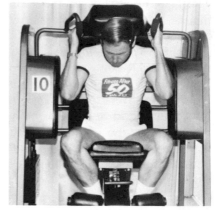

Figures 13–1 and 13–2 above demonstrate abdomen strengthening exercises.

spasm or rebound tenderness are present, referral to a general surgeon is suggested.

The abdominal viscera that may be injured with blunt trauma include most commonly the spleen, often with left lower rib fractures and in athletes with mononucleosis; the liver, often with right lower rib cage or right upper abdominal blunt trauma; and the jejunum, ileum, colon, duodenum, mesentary, pancreas, stomach, and diaphragm.

Prevention of Abdominal Injuries

Abdominal muscle strengthening exercises as outlined in Chapter 4 (see Figs. 13-1 and 13-2) will afford one protection against abdominal injury.

Genitourinary System

The *kidneys*, although relatively well protected under the rib cage, may be injured either by direct trauma to the flank or by contrecoup injury in which they are violently thrown forward when the athlete stops abruptly. Usually there is pain and tenderness in the flank. In cases of hemorrhage, a flank mass may be left with or without shock. The presence of such a mass, shock, and bloody urine are all indications to seek urologic evaluation. The decision as to which kidneys require surgery and which do not requires the judgment of a skilled genitourinary surgeon.

Ureter injuries, not uncommon with pelvic and vertebral fractures, rarely occur with blunt abdominal trauma.

Lower abdominal blunt trauma may result in contusion or rupture of the *bladder*. Rupture with escape of blood and urine into the peritoneal cavity is more common if the bladder is full at the time of trauma. Retroperitoneal rupture and leakage of blood and urine are more common with fractures of the pelvis. Cystography will establish the rupture and need for geni-

155

tourinary referral, as rupture with urine and blood leakage is usually best managed with exploration and repair.

The male *urethra* is divided into two parts. The front part is mobile and, therefore, rarely injured. The posterior part, including the membranous urethra and the prostatic urethra, is susceptible to blunt injury, especially with pelvic fractures. Mild trauma may produce obstruction and inability to void, while severe trauma causes tissue damage, hematoma formation, and escape of blood or urine or both. Urethography and panendoscopy best demonstrate the pathology and are best directed by a genitourinary surgeon.

Because the *female urethra* is short and mobile, injury is uncommon. Blunt trauma from cycling and gymnastics rarely result in contusion, laceration, or frank disruption.

The *scrotum* and its contents are very susceptible to blunt trauma, as it lies in an exposed location. It should be carefully protected by appropriate equipment in all contact sports. Contusion is the most common injury and can usually be alleviated by ice and elevation. If there is a mass or suggestion of continued bleeding, or if the athlete has a single gonad (a relative contraindication to contact sports), urologic examination is advised.

Chapter 14

Upper Limb Injuries

Your shoulder has the widest range of motion of any joint in your body. Your shoulder is a complex region consisting of the shoulder joint, its capsular support, and the dynamic muscle groups that control the motion of your shoulder (see Figs. 14-1 to 14-3).

Your shoulder plays an integral role in virtually all athletic activities. The role of your upper extremity in running or skating sports is both power and balance. Many sports that involve the throwing motion (pitching in baseball, quarterbacking in football, the serve and overhead in tennis, and the freestyle and butterfly motions of swimming) demand far more of your shoulder than nature originally intended.

While your upper extremity is a critical end organ in the act of throwing, the coordination and balance of the rest of your body is vital. An inflamed great toe or low back pain may disrupt the athlete's body muscular rhythm and alter throwing biomechanics, leading to shoulder injury.

Fimrite popularized the Dizzy Dean Syndrome, the situation of creating a second injury by favoring a prior one. Dizzy Dean, an overpowering right-handed pitcher for the St. Louis Cardinals in the 1930s, was struck on the left foot by a line drive and broke his big toe in the 1937 All-Star Game. Two weeks later, he attempted to return to pitching, wearing a splint and an oversized shoe. By favoring his injured toe, he altered his natural pitching motion, which led to a shoulder injury eventually diagnosed as an inflammation of the deltoid muscle at its insertion on the humerus. He had been a more than 30-game winner, but he was to win only 16 games before premature retirement four years later. Smokey Joe Wood is another baseball pitcher who suffered a similar fate. Known for his fastball, and winner of 34 games in 1912, Wood fell while fielding a ground ball in the spring of 1913 and sustained a fractured thumb on his pitching hand. He, too, attempted to return too soon and, with an altered delivery, incurred a shoulder injury that claimed his career.

Figure 14–1

BONES, LIGAMENTS, CAPSULE AND BURSA
OF THE SHOULDER

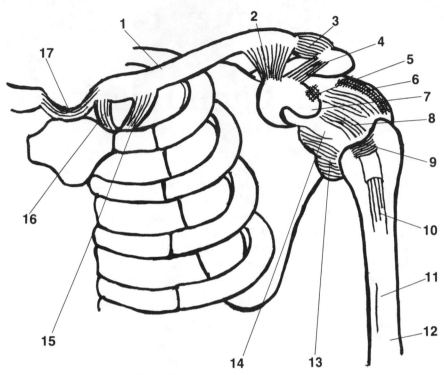

1. Clavicle
2. Coracoclavicular Ligament
3. Acromioclavicular Ligament
4. Coracoacromial Ligament
5. Subacromial Bursa
6. Subacoracoid Bursa
7. Coracoid Process
8. Coracohumeral Ligament
9. Transverse Humeral Ligament
10. Biceps Tendon
11. Bicipital Groove
12. Humerus
13. Capsular Ligament
14. Synovial Capsule
15. Costoclavicular Ligament
16. Anterior Sternoclavicular Ligament
17. Interclavicular Ligament
18. Clavicle

Figure 14–2

ANTERIOR MUSCLES OF THE SHOULDER

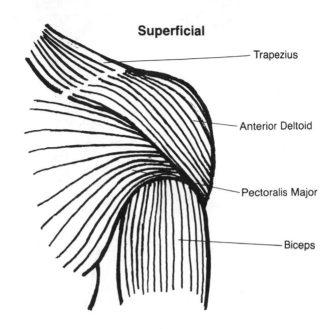

Superficial

Trapezius

Anterior Deltoid

Pectoralis Major

Biceps

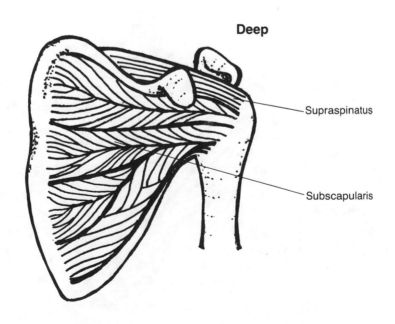

Deep

Supraspinatus

Subscapularis

Figure 14–3

POSTERIOR MUSCLES OF THE SHOULDER

Superficial

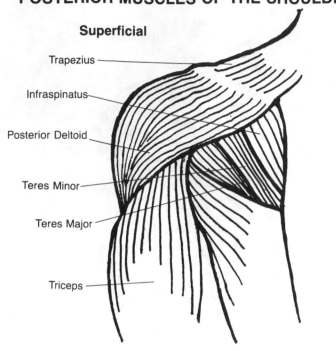

Trapezius

Infraspinatus

Posterior Deltoid

Teres Minor

Teres Major

Triceps

Deep

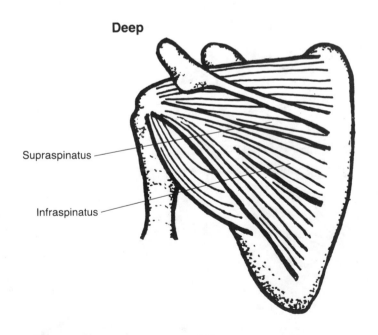

Supraspinatus

Infraspinatus

Thus, when evaluating a painful shoulder, one must be cognizant of the fact that problems with other areas of the body may be a contributing factor.

Acute (Macrotrauma) Shoulder Injuries

Most acute shoulder injuries are the result of a single, major, abrupt force. You are able to recall the specific incident, and diagnosis is usually obvious by examination and x-rays taken in two planes at 90° to each other. Deformity is common, and pain is almost always present. These lesions include sprains, dislocations, and fractures that occur about the shoulder girdle.

Sprains, subluxations (partial dislocation), and dislocations are essentially a continuum of the same process: a variable degree of injury to the ligaments and adjacent soft tissues that normally provide for the integrity of a joint.

Dislocation is characterized by major (75 to 100%) ligamentous disruption, and sprain with minimal ligamentous tear (less than 25%) with a stable joint. There is moderate sensitivity to palpation over the injured area and mild to moderate swelling. The initial treatment, as with sprains elsewhere, is ice for the first 12 to 24 hours, heat thereafter, rest, and appropriate strapping of the area for 1 to 3 weeks. After all pain is gone, an appropriate exercise program should be undertaken. Return to competition should be delayed until strength in the injured shoulder equals that in the noninjured shoulder. Throughout the treatment period, a conplementary program for continued general conditioning should be maintained.

The shoulder joint itself and where the clavicle meets the shoulder and the breastbone are the sites where sprains, subluxations, dislocations, and fractures occur in the shoulder. Most injuries to the clavicle-shoulder articulation occur secondary to a direct fall on the elbow or outstretched hand, resulting in a directed force along the extremity to the acromioclavicular joint.

While the initial treatment is the same as for a sprain (a sling shoulder immobilizer with appropriate compressive padded dressing), referral to an orthopedist is recommended. In Table 14-1, the various sports are ranked according to risk of shoulder injury.

Of all acute injuries to the glenohumeral joint, 98% occur to the anterior portion. This is partly because the anatomy has less support anteriorly, but also because most injuries occur with the arm abducted and externally rotated (moved away from the body). The arm tackle in football and a moving skier with an entrapped ski pole are common examples. Forces are directed to the posterior joint only when the arm is adducted, internally rotated (moved towards the body), and flexed. Careful determination by examination and x-ray should be carried out to determine if the injury is anterior or posterior. If there is a dislocation or if the athlete describes the

Table 14-1
Injury to

	Hand/Wrist Forearm	Elbow	Upper Arm	Shoulder
Archery	L	L	L	L
Automobile racing	M	M	M	M
Baseball	H	H	H	H
Basketball	H	M	M	M
Bicycling	L	L	L	L
Bowling	M	L	L	L
Diving	L	L	L	L
Football	H	H	H	H
Golf	M	L	L	L
Gymnastics	M	M	H	M
Handball	H	M	M	M
Hand gliding	M	M	M	M
Ice hockey	H	H	H	H
Ice-skating	L	L	L	L
Lacrosse	M	M	M	M
Motorcycle racing	H	H	H	H
Racquetball	M	M	M	M
Roller-skating	L	L	L	L
Rowing	L	L	L	L
Rugby	H	H	H	H
Running	M	M	M	M
Skiing	M	M	M	M
Soccer	L	L	L	L
Squash	M	M	M	M
Swimming	L	H	M	H
Tennis	M	M	M	M
Volleyball	M	M	M	M
Water skiing	M	M	M	M
Weight lifting	M	M	M	M
Wrestling	H	H	H	H

L = low risk of injury   M = moderate risk of injury   H = high risk of injury

shoulder as popping forward and then back into place (subluxation), ortho-pedic referral is advised. When pain only in the anterior or posterior gleno-humeral joint is described, a sprain is the diagnosis. Treatment consists of immobilization for 7 to 14 days either in a shoulder immobilizer or in a sling, wrapped with elasticized bandages. General conditioning exercises and a postinjury rehabilitation program similar to that for an acro-mioclavicular sprain are recommended.

Injury to the sternoclavicular joint usually results from forces that drive the shoulder girdle forward while thrusting the clavicle toward the sternum.

They are similarly classified as sprain, subluxation, dislocation, and fracture. All but the sprain should have orthopedic evaluation. The sprain is treated with a sling until pain subsides, and with the other measures for sprains previously discussed. The return to competition follows the same guidelines as for acromioclavicular sprains.

Overuse (Microtrauma) Injuries

There has been a recent increase in the troublesome overuse syndromes involving the shoulder region. The painful pitcher's shoulder has plagued participants, trainers, and team physicians for years, and now similar chronic injuries are frequently seen among recreational, as well as competitive, swimmers and tennis players. Insidious in onset and only annoying in the initial stages, overuse injuries relentless increase in intensity and severity may eventually totally disable the athlete.

An overuse syndrome is defined as a chronic inflammatory condition caused by repeated microtrauma from a repetitious activity. Such injuries may be classified as (1) first degree, those causing pain only after activity; (2) second degree, those producing pain during participation and after, but not enough pain to interfere with performance; and (3) third degree, those resulting in disabling pain both during and after participation.

Overuse syndromes around the shoulder area are particularly common in throwing sports, swimming, and tennis. To appreciate the spectrum of injuries that may occur in throwing, one must comprehend the mechanism of this strenuous activity. During the initial cocking motion, the arm is brought back into abduction, extension, and external rotation. Consequently, the middle and posterior aspects of the deltoid are functioning as well as the infraspinatous and teres minor to produce rotation. The trapezius and rhomboids contribute to scapular elevation and adduction. During the cocking stage, the posterior capsule is relaxed, whereas the anterior capsule, subscapularis, and pectoral muscles are passively elongating. The next stage of throwing consists of the acceleration phase, in which the arm begins to move forward again, often preceded by a forward rotation of the trunk. During this activity, the anterior muscle groups, particularly the subscapularis, pectorals, and anterior deltoid, are contracting while still lengthening (eccentrically). The biceps muscle also may contract, increasing tension on the tendon within the bicipital groove, which is externally rotated. It is during this early part of the acceleration phase that the anterior capsule is particularly stretched. As the arm comes forward into the final follow-through position, the posterior capsule and external rotators are relaxed and passively stretched. Anteriorly, the capsular ligaments can become attenuated and allow the humeral head to sublux and even dislocate. Succen contractures of the subscapularis and pectoral muscles can produce tearing and rupture of these muscular ten-

163

dinous units. Impingement can occur anteriorly around the coracoid, and posteriorly as the humeral head abuts the glenoid. The bicipital tendon and suptraspinatous tendon can abut the acromion and coracoacromial ligament, producing impingement syndromes. Small tears in the rotator-cuff muscles, as well as chronic subdeltoid bursitis, frequently follow as a result of these repeated impingements. Hypertrophic bony changes may occur along the inferior aspect of the glenoid, as well as chronic subluxation of the biceps tendon from its groove. Since the acromioclavicular joint contributes to abduction and rotation, chronic degenerative changes at that site may produce pain, felt over the top of the shoulder and radiating both anteriorly and posteriorly. It is obvious that the throwing mechanism is very complex and can cause symptoms and injuries in numerous areas.

The overhead serve is quite similar to a throwing motion and produces many of the same injuries as are seen in pitchers.

A condition referred to as swimmer's shoulder is seen in freestyle and butterfly-stroke swimmers. These strokes produce repeated impingement of the greater tuberosity under the coracoacromial arch. As the arm is brought forward into abduction, forward flexion, and internal rotation, the region of the supraspinatous tendon and biceps tendon in its groove sustain repeated trauma under the acromion and coracoacromial ligament. As the arm is then pulled down into an adducted position in the follow-through motion, the blood flow into the distal portion of the rotator cuff and biceps tendon is impeded by the pressure of the humeral head from below.

The diagnosis of overuse shoulder syndromes is best carried out by a sports medicine orthopedist. A careful history is perhaps the most important step in diagnosis. Previous training programs and prior history of shoulder subluxation or acromioclavicular-joint separation should be obtained. Such injuries are often experienced early in the season or during periods of double-session workouts. Repeated examinations are often necessary to localize the site of the tenderness and to detect relative weaknesses in the rotator-muscle groups. A neurologic examination is needed to rule out the various nerve compression syndromes. Vascular problems must also be considered. Routine x-rays and, occasionally, special views are necessary, and degenerative changes must also be ruled out. Shoulder arthrograms may be indicated when a rotator-cuff tear is suspected (Figure 14-4). An enlarged capsule may also be noted on arthrography in a chronic subluxing shoulder. Additional x-ray studies should be done only after a careful examination has been performed to determine the exact site of tenderness, the arc of motion that produces pain, and the presence of any specific weakness.

Treatment of overuse syndromes is directed at reducing inflammation and altering training and performance techniques to prevent recurrence. First- and second-degree injuries that produce pain primarily after participation and are not disabling should be treated promptly to prevent their progression. Proper warm-up exercises prior to participation, and ice fol-

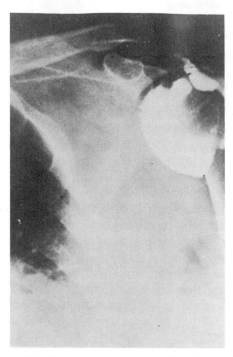

Figure 14–4. This X-ray shows a rotator cuff tear in the shoulder.

lowing competition, may help to relieve the inflammatory changes. Oral anti-inflammatory agents such as aspirin or one of the other nonsteroidal medications are often helpful. Reducing the amount of time throwing, swimming, or serving may help to control the pain. It is essential to review the problem with the coach, since minor changes in technique, such as the amount of elevation in the arm in throwing or swimming, may be necessary. Since these injuries frequently lead to contracture and muscle weakness, it is important to seek these problems out and correct them with flexibility exercises and specific strengthening programs. Isokinetic machines are very helpful in detecting relative weakness in the shoulder.

Third-degree injuries usually require a period of rest. During this time, conditioning programs for the other areas of the body may be continued. Local injections of steroids into the involved areas have been helpful in some cases. However, it must be remembered that these injections produce local tissue necrosis and weaken the structures for at least two weeks. During that time, no vigorous participation should be undertaken. Other modalities can be used to reduce inflammation, especially ultrasound and diatherym. Since recurrence of these injuries is very common, the participant must have full range of motion, equal strength, and be free of pain before returning to competition. Since both coordination and endurance

165

are essential in these sports, it is important to progress slowly to avoid future difficulties.

Shoulder Exercise

Although tissue contractures due to tissue scarring may occur after injury to any joint in the body, your shoulder is especially prone to this problem, and recovery is painfully slow. To help guard against this problem, within pain-free limits, the primary shoulder movements of abduction and external rotation are begun almost immediately after injury. The non-gravity pendular movements allow free range of motion to the shoulder, preventing joint contractures and rotator cuff atrophy (the frozen shoulder syndrome). When pain has subsided, the shoulder should be fully reconditioned with resistance exercises until strength and range of motion equate with the uninjured shoulder. Some of the best shoulder-strengthening exercises include push-ups, the shoulder shrug (deltoids) (Fig. 14-5), lateral raise (deltoids) (Fig. 14-6), overhead press (deltoids and triceps) (Fig. 14-7a, b), overhead pulldown (latissimus dorsi and biceps) (Fig. 14-8), shoulder abduction (deltoids, trapezius) (Fig. 14-9), and decline press (chest, shoulders, triceps) (Fig. 14-10).

Upper Arm Injuries

Depending on the nature of the sport, varied stresses and trauma are directed to your upper arm. Collision and contact sports may subject this region to crushing blows, resulting in contusion (bruise) or fracture of the humerus. The throwing sports and gymnastics subject your upper arm to severe stresses that may lead to sprains and strains.

The treatment of contusions, sprains, and strains is as previously discussed (RICE, p. 118). Two conditions unique to this area bear mention, however. Athletes involved in the throwing motion (baseball pitchers, football quarterbacks, tennis players, javelin throwers) may develop an inflammation of the origin of the biceps tendon. An ache or frank pain is experienced in the anterior and medial aspect of the shoulder, and point tenderness is present over the upper biceps tendon. This condition (bicipital tendonitis) is treated by a program as for tendinitis elsewhere (RICE) followed by deep heat or ultrasound and, finally, after all pain has subsided, resistive biceps exercises (Fig. 14-11).

Rupture (third-degree strain) of the biceps muscle is an injury most often seen in gymnasts involved in a power move. The tear usually occurs near the origin of the biceps muscle. You will usually hear a snap and experience intense pain as if shot in the upper arm with a bullet. A bulge will often be seen in the lower biceps muscle from the rolled-up torn portion of the muscle. Treatment should consist of RICE plus a trip to your orthopedist, as surgical repair is usually necessary.

166

Fractures of the upper arm usually occur as a result of a direct blow or fall. Fractures may produce serious injury to the radial nerve, with resultant wrist drop. The axillary artery may also be severed. When deformity is present, a fracture is virtually always present, and immediate medical evaluation is essential to avoid permanent neurological or vascular injury to the arm. When deformity is not present after a blow or fall on the upper arm, but pain does not subside after several days of RICE treatment, you should suspect an impacted or nondisplaced fracture. X-rays will confirm or eliminate your suspicions.

Elbow Injuries

Your elbow is a hinge joint involving three bones: the lower end of the humerus, the upper end of the radius, and olecranon and coronoid processes of the ulna. The radius can rotate around the ulna, allowing for supination (palm up) and pronation (palm down) of the forearm. The annular, ulnar, and radial collateral ligaments and articular capsule maintain joint stability (Fig. 14-12). The biceps, triceps, and brachialis muscles allow the joint to function (Fig. 14-13).

Your elbow, because of its lack of padding, is very vulnerable to acute injury in collision sports. Contusions, sprains, and strains are all common, and the sports of greatest risk are enumerated in Table 14-1. Hyperextension injuries are quite common in competitive and recreational activities. Subluxation (partial dislocation), dislocation, or fracture may occur as a result of direct trauma. As with the shoulder, subluxation, dislocation, or fracture of the elbow should have orthopedic evaluation. Sprains and strains should initially receive the RICE treatment.

Recurrent microtrauma is the cause of chronic overuse elbow injuries such as tennis elbow. Frequently seen in tennis players, this condition is common to all racket-sport players and virtually all recreational activities that involve the arms. The primary site of pain and point tenderness is in the region of the extensor muscle origin from the lateral epicondyle. It is now agreed that the basic pathology is an inflammation of the aponeurosis overlying the extensor carpi radialis and the extensor communis. Overuse and overload (often aggravated by improper stroke production), usually associated with a lack of appropriate preconditioning, is the mechanical cause. Prevention, therefore, includes appropriate advice regarding conditioning and proper technique.

The initial treatment of tennis elbow is rest, ice for the first 24 hours, heat thereafter, and oral anti-inflammatory medication. If symptoms persist, a single injection of local steroid and anesthetic into the area of point tenderness may be tried. If an injection is made, the arm should not be strenuously used for the next two weeks due to the steroid's weakening effect on ligaments and tendons.

Figure 14–5

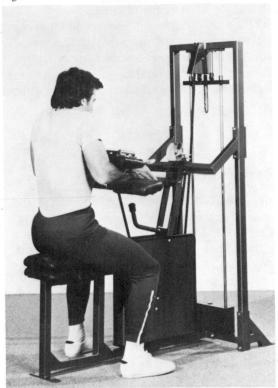

Figure 14–6

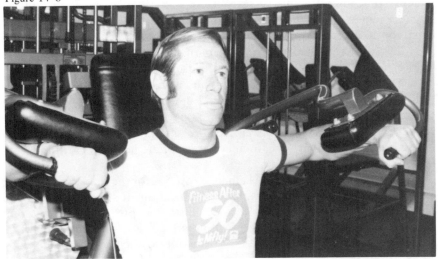

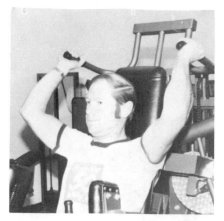

Figure 14–7a

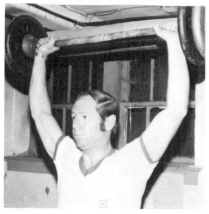

Figure 14–7b

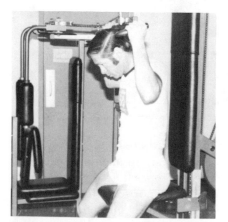

Figure 14–8

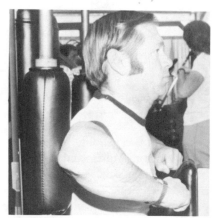

Figure 14–9

Figures 14–5 to 14–10 demonstrate
various shoulder strengthening exercises.

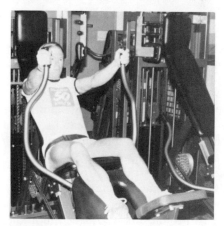

Figure 14–10

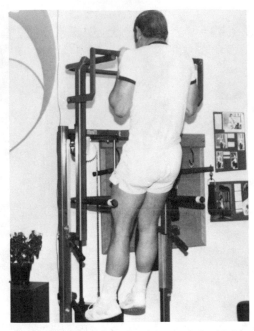

Figure 14–11. Dr. Cantu demonstrates a resistive biceps exercise.

Rehabilitation should include flexibility exercises to assure full range of elbow motion and isotonic and isometric exercises to maintain maximum forearm muscular strength. It may also be appropriate to direct attention toward technique and equipment, such as size and weight of the racket, tension of strings, and circumference of handle grip. While a lighter-weight racket, lower-tension strings, and a larger handle-grip may help, the best solution is to combine these changes with a fiberglass or composite racket that dampens vibrations.

In chronic subacute situations (a common occurrence among tennis players who will play through injury), the use of an elbow brace or nonelastic band distal to the elbow, which decreases the excursion and stress on the extensor origin, may be extremely helpful. As one who played in many tournaments during an 8-month bout with this condition, I know that the elbow brace can make the difference between having to stop and being able to continue playing. If the condition has persisted for a year or more without any signs of improvement, orthopedic referral for consideration of surgical intervention may be appropriate.

The second most common overuse elbow injury occurs from throwing. The same sports as discussed with the shoulder may produce elbow injury, as the forces moving through the shoulder in throwing or other athletic action are extended distally through the arm to the elbow. The acceleration and follow-through (the final phases of throwing) place tremendous stress

Figure 14–12

BONES, LIGAMENTS, CAPSULE AND BURSA OF THE ELBOW

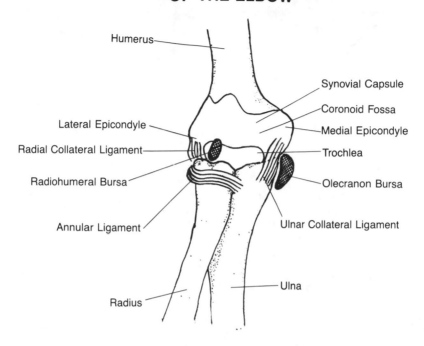

Figure 14–13

MUSCLES OF THE ELBOW, LATERAL ASPECT

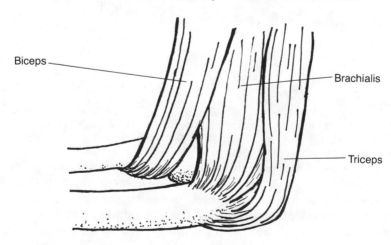

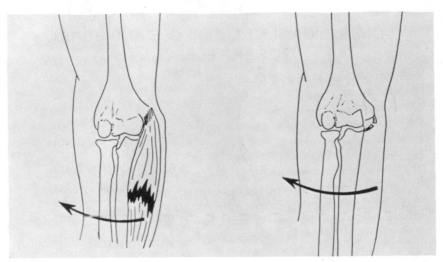

Figure 14–14. Left, a flexor muscle tear. Right, a medial collateral ligament rupture. Reproduced with permission from *Sports Medicine in Primary Care* by Robert C. Cantu, M.D., © 1982 D.C. Heath and Company.

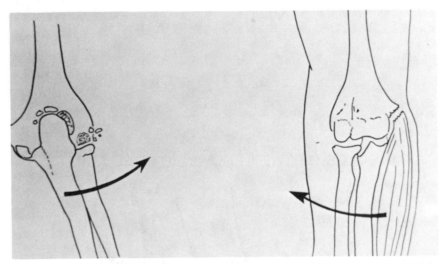

Figure 14–15. Left, ulnar traction spur and medial collateral ligament attenuation. Right, medial epicondylar avulsion fracture. Reproduced with permission from *Sports Medicine in Primary Care* by Robert C. Cantu, M.D. © 1982 D.C. Heath and Company.

on the elbow. The *medial* side of the elbow is stretched and the *lateral* side is compressed, as is the *olecranon* and *distal humerus*. In the follow-through motion, extreme compressive forces are generated in the concavity of the olecranon by athletes who perform repetitive throwing motion (Figs. 14-14 and 14-15).

Bony avulsions, injuries to the flexor mass, ulnar nerve inflammation secondary to repetitive stretch and/or subluxation in the ulnar groove, and spurs on the medial edge of the olecranon are the most common problems occurring on the medial side of the elbow from throwing. All of these must be considered, and in the young athlete frank avulsion of the medial epicondyle must be considered as well.

The compressive forces on the lateral side of the elbow between the radial head and the capitellum may result in a shearing action on the elbow joint resulting in damage to the articular cartilage with progressive fragmentation and formation of bone chips (Fig. 14-16).

In the skeletally immature athlete with open growth centers, the compressive lateral forces may lead to abnormalities of growth and resultant deformity. "Little League elbow" is an example (Fig. 14-17). While it is impossible to define chronologic age limits as to when a young athlete with open epiphyses with active growth potential should and should not pitch, since this is related to individual skeletal development and maturation, the Little League restrictions for limited pitching are strongly recommended. Clearly, the greater the number of innings pitched by a youth with open epiphyses, the more likely the development of elbow impairment and ultimate restriction of an athletic career. The curveball and screwball, because of the snap motion, produce the greatest stress on the elbow and should be thrown only by the skeletally mature athlete.

The treatment of any of the throwing injuries, whether in the baseball pitcher, gymnast, or tennis player, should involve orthopedic referral if any of the various bone pathologies are visible on x-ray. If ulnar nerve injury

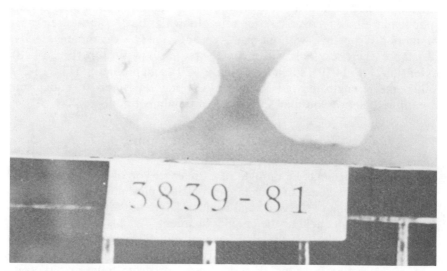

Figure 14–16. Bone chips. Reproduced with permission from *Sports Medicine in Primary Care* by Robert C. Cantu, M.D. © 1982 D.C. Heath and Company.

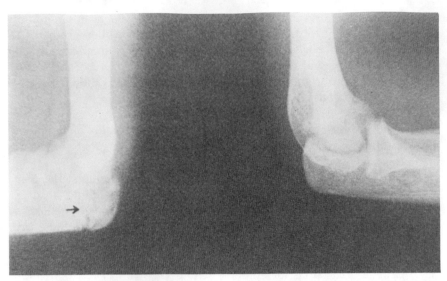

Figure 14–17. Little league elbow. Reproduced with permission from *Sports Medicine in Primary Care* by Robert C. Cantu, M.D. © 1982 D.C. Heath and Company.

is present with numbness of the fifth finger and lateral half of the fourth finger, usually without hand-muscle weakness or atrophy in the early stages, neurosurgical referral is suggested.

Elbow Exercises

During the initial RICE treatment of elbow injuries, exercises should be carried out at the shoulder and wrist joints. Maintaining their strength will speed your elbow recovery. After your elbow has healed and a free range of motion is possible without pain, you are ready to commence active resistance exercises. This will include sets of elbow flexion (Fig. 14-18), extension (Fig. 14-19), supination (Fig. 14-20), and pronation (Fig. 14-21). When the strength in your injured elbow has recovered to equal your noninjured elbow, you may safely return to competition.

Forearm, Wrist, and Hand

The ulna, which may be thought of as an extension of the humerus, and the radius are the bones of your forearm. The radius may be thought of as being an extension of the wrist and is much larger at the wrist. The radius and ulna articulate, held by the annular ligament (Fig. 14-14), at the elbow. This affords the palm-up and palm-down movements of your forearm. Most forearm injuries are either fractures, strains, or abrasions. A Colles fracture of the radius and ulna (Fig. 14-22) results from falling on the outstretched hand or using it to ward off another player. All forearm fractures

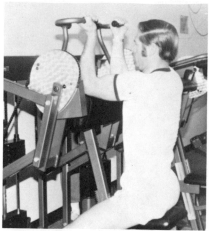

Figure 14–18

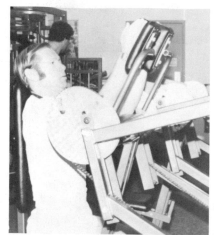

Figure 14–19

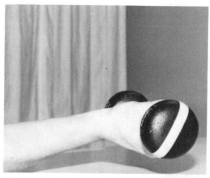

Figure 14–20

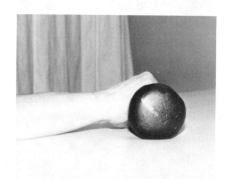

Figure 14–21

Figures 14–18 to 14–20 demonstrate elbow strengthening exercises.

should be seen by an orthopedist. Abrasions, contusions, sprains, and strains can be treated as discussed for the elbow and shoulder.

The wrist (see Fig. 14-23) is composed of the eight carpal and five metacarpal bones. Wrist injuries range from sprains to dislocations that often require open surgical repositioning. Major tendon injuries that may terminate careers also occur. The biomechanical requirement through the wrist and intercarpal joints is greatest in activities requiring a wrist snap and/or turnover intercarpal rotation (swinging at an object, as in baseball, tennis, golf, or lacrosse, or release of an object with sudden wrist action, as in bowling, weight lifting, pole vaulting, javelin, discus, or shot put). The forces generated can lead to strains, dislocations, and carpal fractures. There is no area of sports medicine where accurate diagnosis of an injury is more challenging than at the wrist. Hard-to-see (occult) fractures are

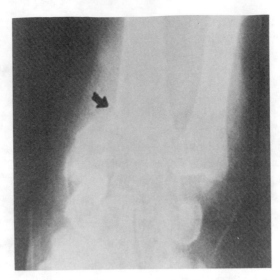

Figure 14–22. A Colles fracture of the radius and ulna. Reproduced with permission from *Sports Medicine in Primary Care* by Robert C. Cantu, M.D. © 1982 D.C. Heath and Company.

Figure 14–23

BONES OF FOREARM, WRIST AND HAND

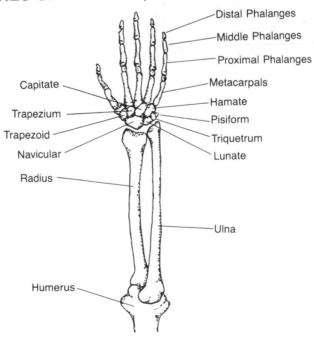

Distal Phalanges

Middle Phalanges

Proximal Phalanges

Capitate

Metacarpals

Hamate

Trapezium

Pisiform

Trapezoid

Triquetrum

Navicular

Lunate

Radius

Ulna

Humerus

common, and it is frequently necessary to obtain comparative views of the noninjured hand, and additional fluoroscopic tomographic or nuclear-scan examinations. If initial x-rays are negative but you do not respond to the initial sprain treatment, additional x-rays should be taken and orthopedic referral made.

The carponavicular joint, the most common site of acute hand fracture, is often not seen on initial x-ray. Malunited or ununited hand bone fracture leads to chronic pain, often requiring surgical intervention for realignment and bone grafting. Treatment of wrist injuries by yourself or by the team physician should be limited to sprains and abrasions. If the symptoms of a strain do not resolve in two weeks, orthopedic referral is prudent.

As with the wrist, sprains, fractures, and dislocations are the most common finger injuries. Orthopedic referral is recommended for all but sprains. Finger fractures that initially appear innocuous may undergo malalignment and malrotation, leading to significant disability. Precise alignment and rotational position and its subsequent maintenance is extremely important in the hand. If this cannot be achieved, early open reduction (repositioning properly) and pin fixation must be considered. The Mallet finger injury, which usually results from a direct blow to the tip of an extended finger, is one of the most common athletic finger injuries. The blow results in a rupture of the tendon at its insertion or avulsion of the tendon with a fragment of bone. Orthopedic referral is advisable, as open reduction may be required.

Finally, in certain sports where a single digital nerve is subjected to continued pressure, as in bowling, baseball, or swinging any object to contact another object, the compressive force may result in the formation of neuromas (tumors made up of nerve substance). Rest, local anesthetics, or steroid injections should be the initial treatment, with prolonged rest as the treatment of preference. Failure to respond should suggest referral to an experienced hand surgeon and/or neurosurgeon for neuroma excision.

Forearm, Wrist, and Hand Exercises

As with other joints, to prevent muscle atrophy and restriction of joint motion, an exercise program should be started as soon as possible following a forearm, wrist, or hand injury. Once pain and swelling have subsided, range of motion progressive to resistance exercises should be started. Ideally, your exercises should be performed in sets of 12 to 15 repetitions twice daily. As strength increases, weight is increased, but not so fast that 12 to 15 repetitions cannot be completed. Return to competition should await regaining full strength.

Excellent exercises to strengthen your forearm, wrist, and hand are shown in Figures 14-24, 25. Dumbbells can be used in flexion (Fig. 14-26) and extension (Fig. 14-27) as well as wrist supination and pronation (Figs. 14-20 and 14-21). In carrying out these exercises, you should stabilize

177

your bent elbow. Other good exercises for the forearm, wrist, and hand include squeezing against a resistance, such as a rubber ball or a spring device (Fig. 14-28).

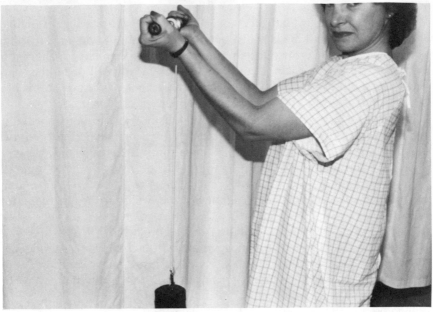

Figure 14–24

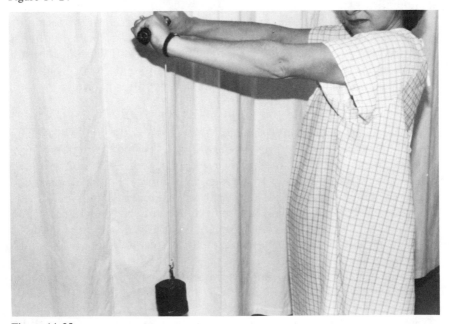

Figure 14–25

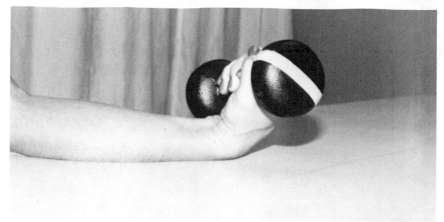

Figure 14–26

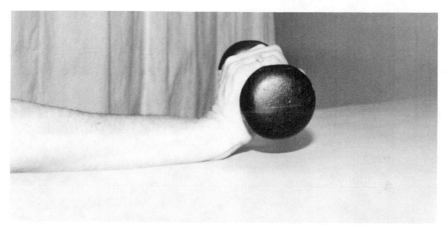

Figure 14–27

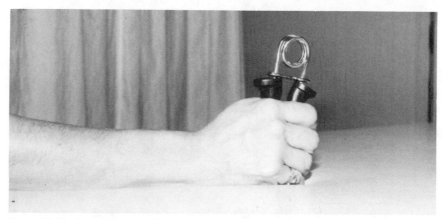

Figure 14–28. A resistive exercise for the forearm, wrist and hand

Chapter 15

Lower Limb Injuries

Pelvis and Hip

The bony pelvis unites the spinal column, through the lumbosacral joint, with the lower extremities, through the hip joints. In addition, the bony pelvis has three joints of its own that can be sites of injury: the two sacro-iliac joints behind and the symphysis pubica in front. Perhaps as important as the joints of the pelvis, however, are the multiple sites of muscle-tendon-unit insertions on the pelvis and in the region of the hip. Many of these muscles are two-joint muscles, with an increased chance of strain or injury, given their increased range of movement (excursion).

The lumbosacral joint is more appropriately discussed with back injuries. The remaining pelvic joints, the sacroiliac and symphysis pubica, are syndesmotic joints (i.e., bound by ligaments) with minimal excursion, which hold the bony elements of the pelvic ring together and allow for stress uptake. Interestingly, we are seeing a new overuse syndrome involving these joints, called osteitis pubica (Fig. 15-1). This is actually an arthritis of the symphysis pubica joint resulting from recurrent microtrauma. It is seen in distance runners and team-sport players who perform on hard surfaces such as synthetic football or soccer turf. It frequently presents as low-grade aching groin pain, with onset after running begins. It is associated with a reactive and often dramatic tightness of the groin muscles, with limited hip abduction (outward movement). Since the pubic region is the site of insertion of both the rectus and abdominis muscles from above and the groin or adductor muscles, osteitis pubica is often mistakenly diagnosed as a strain of these muscles or a tendinitis of their insertions. Plain x-rays are often diagnostic in advanced cases, with irregularity of the pubic margins and bony resorption evident. In less severe or early cases, radiographs may be nondiagnostic. Bone scan can be helpful in diagnosing this condition,

Figure 15–1

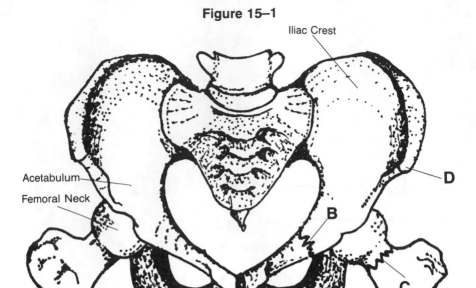

The bony pelvis. Overuse athletic injuries can involve (A) the symphysis pubica: osteitis pubis, (B) stress fractures of the pubic rami, or (C) stress fractures of the neck of the femur. Muscle tendon avulsions can occur at (D) the pelvic brim or (E) icheal rami site of hamstring muscle insertions. Reproduced with permission from *Sports Medicine in Primary Care* by Robert C. Cantu, M.D. © 1982 D.C. Heath and Company.

but recognition is often the result of no more than an index of suspicion and attention to a history of microtrauma.

Treatment begins with relative rest. Sometimes altering the running surface—running on grass instead of pavement, for example—can arrest mild cases. Anti-inflammatory drugs can also be helpful. If one type is unsuccessful, a second or even a third should be tried. Additional physical therapy to stretch and strengthen the groin and abdominal muscles must also be undertaken to rehabilitate the athlete after this injury.

The hip joint is comprised of the articulation of the head of the femur with the deep socket, the acetabulum, of the hip bone. Figures 15-2 and 15-3 depict the many muscles of the hip which move it in.

1. *Flexion:* psoas major, iliacus, tensor, fasciae latae, rectus femoris, sartorius, pectineus, adductor longus, adductor brevis, and gracilis

2. *Extension:* gluteus maximus, hamstring muscles (biceps femoris, semimembranosus, semitendinosus), and adductor magnus

Figure 15–2

LEG MUSCLES, ANTERIOR ASPECT

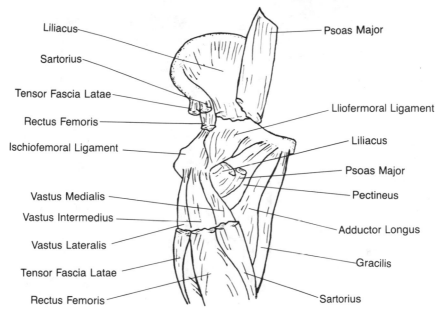

Liliacus

Sartorius

Tensor Fascia Latae

Rectus Femoris

Ischiofemoral Ligament

Vastus Medialis

Vastus Intermedius

Vastus Lateralis

Tensor Fascia Latae

Rectus Femoris

Psoas Major

Lliofermoral Ligament

Liliacus

Psoas Major

Pectineus

Adductor Longus

Gracilis

Sartorius

3. *Adduction:* hamstring muscles, pectineus, gracilis, adductor magnus, adductor longus, adductor brevis, and psoas

4. *Abduction:* tensor fasciae latae, gluteus maximus, gluteus medius, and gluteus minimus

5. *Inward rotation:* gluteus medius, gluteus minimus, tensor fasciae latae, adductor longus, adductor brevis, adductor magnus, and iliopsoas major

6. *Outward rotation:* gluteus maximus, piriformis, obturator externus and obturator internus, the gemelli (superior and inferior), quadratus femoris, sartorius, and adductor magnus

Muscle Strains and Avulsions (Tears)

The most common injuries of the hips and pelvis in athletes are muscle-tendon strains, or even avulsions. The pelvic ring is the site of many muscle insertions: the iliac wing serves as the site of conjoint insertion of the abdominal muscles from above and the gluteal muscles from below; the ischium as the site of origin of the hamstrings; and the pubis and pubic ring anteriorly as the site of insertion of the groin muscles and lesser hip flexors.

Muscle-tendon strain can occur anywhere through the muscle, but adult recreational athletes frequently sustain injury at the muscle-tendon junction, while adolescent athletes can avulse the cartilagenous tendon insertions from the bone itself.

Figure 15–3

THIGH MUSCLES, POSTERIOR ASPECT

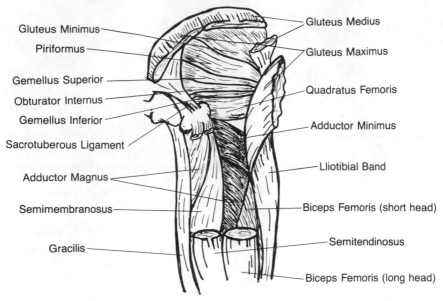

Gluteus Minimus

Piriformus

Gemellus Superior

Obturator Internus

Gemellus Inferior

Sacrotuberous Ligament

Adductor Magnus

Semimembranosus

Gracilis

Gluteus Medius

Gluteus Maximus

Quadratus Femoris

Adductor Minimus

Lliotibial Band

Biceps Femoris (short head)

Semitendinosus

Biceps Femoris (long head)

Injuries to the hips themselves are rare in the recreational athlete. Pain localized to the hip may actually be referred from the back, as a reflection of back disorders. It may also be the result of impingement of adjacent muscle-tendon structures on the hip structures. Hip strains are usually best demonstrated by an inability to circumduct (move circularly around) the thigh.

Trochanteric bursitis can usually be diagnosed by the presence of direct tenderness and, sometimes, swelling over the lateral bony prominence of the hip. Examination of the fascia lata usually demonstrates that it is relatively tight. Management includes relative rest and use of anti-inflammatory medication or even corticosteroid injections. Improving the flexibility and strength of the muscles about the hip and, in particular, of the fascia lata, are most important, however. Onset of hip pain with sports activity can be the first presentation of early degenerative arthritis of the hip. Examination often shows limited rotation of the hips in flexion and extension, often with loss of internal rotation more than external rotation. Radiographs can confirm narrowed joint space and, sometimes, marginal osteophyte (bony outgrowths) formation. The maintenance of hip motion and strength is very important in the early stages of degenerative arthritis of the hip. Exercises such as biking or swimming, rather than running, are usually recommended.

Additionally, persistent hip pain in association with repetitive microtrauma activities, such as running, may reflect a stress fracture of the femoral neck. Plain x-rays may be nondiagnostic, and radioisotope bone scan may be the only way to confirm the diagnosis. If detected early enough, rest alone is sufficient to manage a stress fracture of the hip. Patients should be placed on crutches, and activities such as swimming for a period of 8 to 12 weeks are recommended. Internal fixation or pinning is probably not necessary.

Dancers and gymnasts are especially prone to the snapping hip syndrome. This condition arises from a muscular imbalance as a result of repetitive movements. It usually occurs when the athlete laterally rotates and flexes the hip as part of an exercise or dance routine. Pain and inflammation usually accompany the snapping. After the initial RICE treatment, further rehabilitation focuses on stretching the tight muscles and strengthening the weak ones.

Thigh

The thigh bone, the femur, is the longest and strongest bone in the body. Its configuration permits maximal mobility and support during locomotion. The muscles of the thigh include (see Figs. 15-4 and 15-5):

1. quadriceps (anterior) group—rectus femoris, vastus medialis, intermedius, and lateralis
2. hamstring (posterior) group—biceps femoris, semimembranosus, and semitendinosus
3. adductor (medial) group—adductor longus, magnus, brevis, and psoas
4. abductor (lateral) group—gluteus maximus, medius, minimus

The quadriceps, the most powerful thigh muscle group because of its anterior location, is most vulnerable to direct contusion. A thigh bruise, commonly referred to as a charley horse, should be early subjected to RICE treatment to minimize internal bleeding into the muscle. A charley horse can be minor, moderate, or severe, depending on the relative disability that results. Minor thigh contusions allow full passive and active flexion of the knee and the maintenance of a fully extended knee against resistance. In moderate injuries, while the knee can be passively extended to neutral, complete active or passive flexion of the knee is not possible, but does occur to at least 90°. In severe thigh contusions, there is a dropping of the leg when extension of the elevated leg is attempted and the knee cannot be flexed to 90°. Severe thigh contusions must be treated with great care, and hospitalization may be required to place the extremity at rest. Ice should be applied until passive extension can be maintained; then slow, cautious resumption of motion of the thigh should be commenced.

The feared complication of severe thigh contusion is myositis ossificans, an inflammation of the muscle tissue, with bony deposits. This is actual calcification of the resolving thigh hematoma and may be associated with

185

Figure 15–4

THIGH MUSCLES, QUADRICEPS GROUP

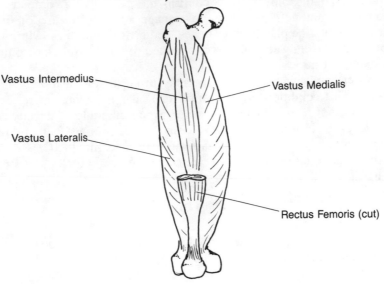

Vastus Intermedius

Vastus Medialis

Vastus Lateralis

Rectus Femoris (cut)

Figure 15–5

THIGH MUSCLES, HAMSTRING GROUP

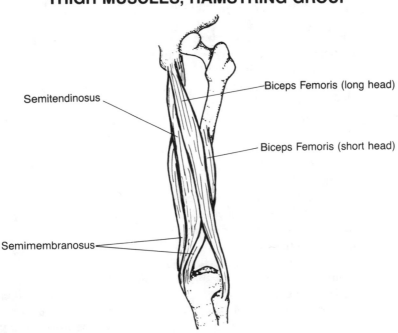

Semitendinosus

Biceps Femoris (long head)

Biceps Femoris (short head)

Semimembranosus

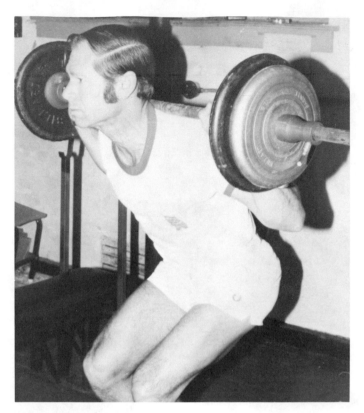

Figure 15–6. Squats.

the early application of heat or excessive rehabilitation of the extremity. It rarely requires surgery, although the disability may last up to a year after injury (Fig. 15-5).

Unsuspected stress fractures of the femoral shaft may also cause thigh or leg pain and should be considered. In addition, referred pain from the lower back and hip region can be confused with local disorders of the leg.

Groin strains represent a tear in the adductor muscle group. Running, jumping, or twisting with external rotation may result in such an injury. Their treatment is as for other strains.

Exercises for the Hip and Thigh

After RICE treatment and after pain has subsided and the full range of motion and flexibility have been restored, active resistance exercises can commence. As discussed previously, the goal is 15 repetitions, progressing from one to three sets once or twice daily. Although squats (Fig. 15-6), hip adduction (Fig. 15-7), and hip abduction (Fig. 15-8) can be done without weights, the machines perhaps best isolate and exercise the hip and thigh muscles (see Figs. 15-9 and 15-10).

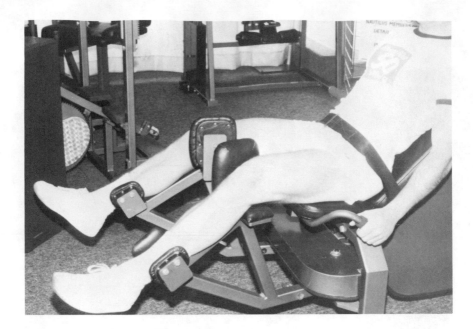

Figure 15–7. Hip adduction.

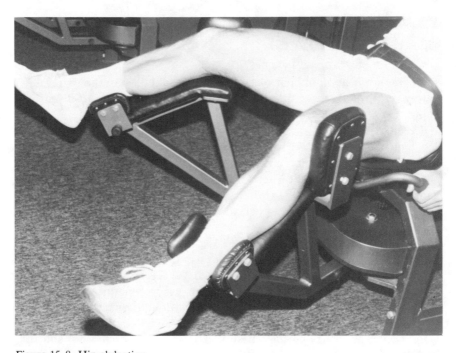

Figure 15–8. Hip abduction.

188

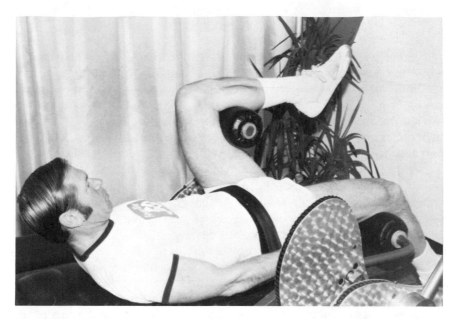

Figure 15–9. Hip and thigh exercise.

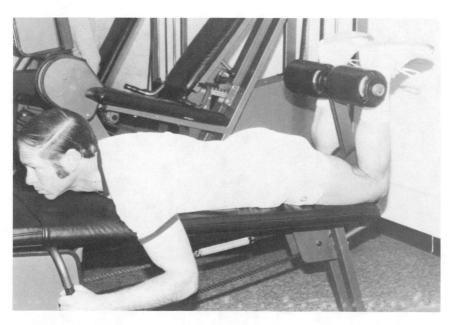

Figure 15–10. Knee flexion exercise.

Knee

The knee is a hinge joint with primarily two motions, flexion and extension. Flexion is accomplished by the biceps femoris, semitendinosus, semimembranosus, gracilis, sartorious, gastrocnemius, popliteus, and plantaris muscles (Fig. 15-10). Extension is executed by the quadriceps, vastus medialis, intermedius, and lateralis, and the rectus femoris (Fig. 15-11). The knee, in flexion only, does allow a slight degree of outward lateral rotation, controlled by the biceps femoris, and medial inward rotation executed by the popliteus, semitendinosus, semimembranosus, sartorius, and gracilis.

Your knee joint is very weak from a bone standpoint and receives its support from the ligaments and muscles that cross it. It is especially weak medially and laterally. The two condyles of the femur articulate with the tibia cushioned by two crescent-shaped cartilages, the medial and lateral menisci. Figure 15-12 shows the many ligaments of your knee, and Figure 15-13 some of the more than 18 bursae located about your knee, each serving to pad and prevent abnormal function.

Being the largest joint in your body and having a shallow, poor bony arrangement with stability being provided by muscular and connective tissue, your knee is especially vulnerable to medial, lateral, and rotational

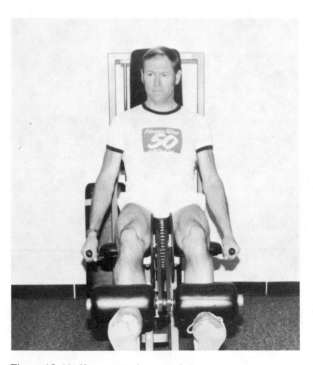

Figure 15–11. Knee extension exercise.

Figure 15–12

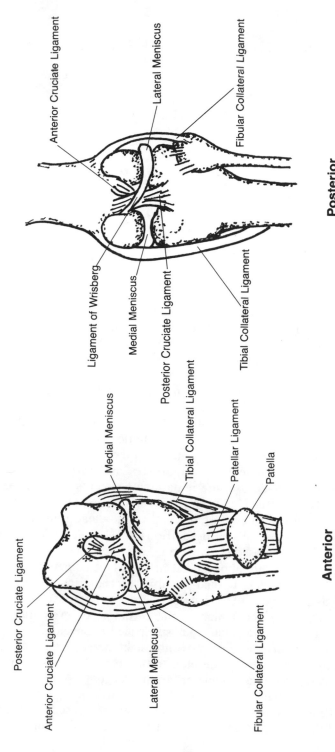

Anterior Cruciate Ligament

Lateral Meniscus

Fibular Collateral Ligament

Ligament of Wrisberg

Medial Meniscus

Posterior Cruciate Ligament

Tibial Collateral Ligament

Posterior

Medial Meniscus

Tibial Collateral Ligament

Patellar Ligament

Patella

Posterior Cruciate Ligament

Anterior Cruciate Ligament

Lateral Meniscus

Fibular Collateral Ligament

Anterior

KNEE LIGAMENTS

191

Figure 15–13

MAJOR BURSA OF THE KNEE

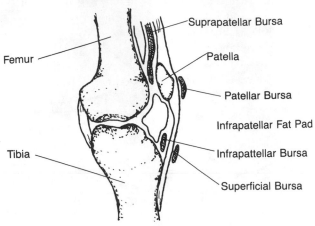

forces. Knee disorders are the most frequently encountered problems in most sports. In contact sports, cutting injuries or direct-impact injuries can cause severe, and frequently disabling, knee injuries. Even in running or dancing, however, knee problems can lead the list. While assessment of knee injuries can often be difficult, even for the knee expert, classifying the injuries or problems into three different types is helpful: ligamentous internal derangements, and derangements of the extensor mechanism. Combinations of two or even three of these disorders can occur together. For example, a cutting injury that tears the anterior cruciate ligament may initially appear to be of minor importance after the initial pain and swelling have resolved, and the athlete may actually resume sports in a short time. However, with continued use, the remaining ligaments of the knee may undergo progressive stretching to the point where the knee may begin to give way, reflecting a rotatory instability. Straight-ahead running may still be possible without any problem. In addition to the knee's beginning to give way, however, the increased laxity of the knee increases the chance of a tear developing in the lateral or medial meniscus or, sometimes, in both. Finally, the ligamentous laxity and possible associated meniscal tear can affect the fit and excursion of the patella in its femoral groove. As a result, chondromalacia patella (softening of the cartilage) or even subluxation (partial dislocation) of the patella may subsequently develop.

Similarly, a previous knee injury, with a slight increase in general laxity and a silent meniscal tear, may develop, rather typical symptoms of chondromalacia patella when a running program is begun.

Recently, the growing use of the fiberoptic arthroscope as an aid in examining the interior of the knee has dramatically increased the diagnostic acumen and the therapeutic collection of the sports physician. Getting a careful history and complete physical examination is still important, and this new diagnostic technique has dramatically impoved our ability to assess and treat knee injuries in athletes. The knee is one of the most difficult joints to assess, and I urge you to indulge in no self-diagnosis if pain and swelling do not quickly subside after injury, or if the knee buckles or locks. A thorough examination by an orthopedist is recommended.

Much remains to be learned about the combination of the ligamentous injuries and the resultant laxities of the knee. The most recent classification divides these ligamentous instabilities of the knee into straight instabilities and rotatory instabilities. The straight instabilities include valgus, varus, anterior, and posterior instabilities.

Valgus instability, reflecting tears of the medial collateral ligament complex, usually results from a blow to the outer side of the knee. This is a relatively benign derangement, and operative repair is no longer considered unless a complete third-degree tear with associated injury of the posterior capsule has occurred. Similarly, varus instability of the knee is usually well tolerated and will generally respond to conservative treatment. Isolated anterior and posterior instabilities are rarely encountered.

Of the rotatory instabilities, most are presently thought to be a reflection of a tear of the internal cruciate ligaments.

A high index of suspicion, especially for the possibility of anterior cruciate injury, must be entertained when the knee injury occurs in sports in which the athlete recalls a sensation of a pop in the knee, acute onset of swelling in the knee, or a sensation of giving way of the knee or transient instability.

The present approach to knee injuries with an associated bloody swelling within the knee requires careful orthopedic assessment, often under general anesthesia, and often by arthroscopy. This incidence of major internal derangement is high in this condition.

A chronic instability, which may have resulted from injury months or years earlier, is seen much more frequently. In such situations, particularly in the recreational athlete, a thorough rehabilitative program of exercises to restore the strength of the hamstrings, and the possible adjunctive use of a brace such as the Lenox-Hill derotational brace, may be sufficient to allow ongoing activities and prevent further deterioration of the knee. Surgical reconstruction of the chronic unstable knee should be attempted only when there is a progressive functional loss.

Derangements of the knee cartilage are the most common internal derangements of the knee. A young athlete may present a locked knee because of an acute cartilage tear, but cartilage tears in the recreational adult are usually of the degenerative type, which usually present more insidiously. These tears are often evident as a low-grade ache in the back of the knee with or without associated swelling and sometimes with an associated catch in the knee with activity. True locking is rare, and it can be due to a loose body or fragment instead of a meniscal derangement.

Both the assessment and management of internal derangements have been revolutionized by the arthroscope. In most centers, arthroscopy has replaced arthrography (injecting dye inside the knee joint and taking x-rays) in assessing internal derangements, particularly with the refinement of microsurgical techniques under arthroscopic control. Most internal derangements in the adult athlete can now be diagnosed and treated with the arthroscopic technique. A knee problem that does not respond to exercise techniques to restore motion and strength and that continues to suggest a derangement of the articular mechanics of the knee is now usually considered for arthroscopic evaluation. Arthroscopy can be done under local anesthesia on an outpatient basis, and repair of many of the conditions encountered—such as the presence of loose bodies or tears of the meniscus—can be effected under the same anesthesia, using separate small puncture wounds in the knee and small grasping and cutting instruments.

Extensor mechanism problems are the most commonly encountered knee problems in the recreational athlete. Derangement of the patella (knee cap), patellar tendon, or quadriceps tendon may occur separately, or in combination. Swimmer's knee, runner's knee, jumper's knee, or biker's knee are terms applied to derangements of the extensor mechanism.

The history is usually diagnostic. A low-grade aching pain, usually activity-related, is described and localized to the front of the knee. Transient episodes of giving way are often described, but these are not followed by locking or swelling of the knee, and immediate resumption of motion is possible. Pain with stair-climbing is often noted, as well as stiffness or aching occurring with prolonged sitting in one position, as with driving or sitting in a movie. There is often an additional history of change in intensity or physical activity preceding the onset of symptoms. Most derangements of the extensor mechanism are overuse injuries and are the result of the recurrent microtrauma of running or jumping.

Examination will often reveal one or more elements of associated anatomic malalignment of the lower extremity, such as leg-length discrepancy, pigeon toe, high arch, or flat foot. Examination of the muscle-tendon units will often reveal a relatively tight and weak quadriceps muscle, with the vastus lateralis stronger than the vastus medialis and associated tight fascia lata. The end result, again, is a tendency toward lateral tracking of the patella in its groove with resultant asymmetric wearing of the articular surface of the patella and, in severe cases, frank lateral luxation (dislocation) of the patella. Table 15-1 outlines the associated risk factors that should be anticipated in an overuse injury such as chondromalacia patella (degeneration of the cartilage of the knee cap).

Knee Exercises

Early on, and in relatively mild cases, restoring the balance of strength and flexibility of the muscles of the lower extremity—especially of the quadriceps itself—may be sufficient to alleviate symptoms. A program of

Table 15-1*

Associated Risk Factors in an Overuse Injury

Training errors, including abrupt changes in intensity, duration, or frequency of training.

Musculotendinous imbalance of strength, flexibility, or bulk.

Anatomic malalignment of the lower extremities, including difference in leg lengths, abnormalities of rotation of the hips, position of the knee cap, and bow legs, knock knees, or flat feet.

Footwear: improper fit, inadequate impact-absorbing material, excessive stiffness of the sole, and/or insufficient support of hindfoot.

Running surface: concrete pavement versus asphalt versus running track versus dirt or grass.

Associated disease state of the lower extremity, including arthritis, poor circulation, old fracture, or other injury.

---

*Reproduced with permission from *Sports Medicine in Primary Care* by Robert C. Cantu, M.D. © 1982 D.C. Heath and Company.

---

general lower-extremity stretching exercises, especially for the quadriceps, fascia lata, and hamstrings, and a program of static straight-leg-raising strengthening exercises of the quadriceps should be followed. These exercises are done with the leg in full extension, with weight boot or ankle weights, lifted from the hip while the opposite hip and knee are flexed. This must be a progressive resistive program with increase in the amount of weights lifted as strength improves. A resistance of at least 12 pounds must be obtained, lifted in three sets of 10 repetitions, before symptoms are usually relieved. In the average-sized adult, a level of 18 to 25 pounds of resistance, maintained for at least six months, successfully relieves patello-femoral symptoms more than 90% of the time.

Additional measures to relieve patellofemoral symptoms may include the use of orthotics (foot supports) in both street and athletic shoes to prevent associated pronation (inward movement of the foot); in severe cases, knee braces may also be useful by helping to distribute the extensor forces across the knee. If these steps do not relieve symptoms over a period of at least six months, surgery may be necessary.

We prefer to call this condition patellofemoral stress syndrome rather than chondromalacia patella, unless frank fissuring and deterioration of the articular surface of the patella can be confirmed either by arthroscopy or arthrotomy. In many cases, these symptoms are associated with simple mild softening of the articular cartilage. Intervention with exercises or even surgery in this disorder must be truly preventative to be helpful. If this disorder has progressed to the point where extensive deterioration of the articular cartilage of the patella has already occurred, results of subsequent management are usually poor.

Recent interest in debridement or filing down roughened cartilage of the undersurface of the patella (chondroplasty) has developed because such debridement can now be done using power instruments under arthroscopic control. While these techniques may give symptomatic relief, every attempt must be made to restore the proper tracking of the patella in its groove, since these degenerative changes are secondary to the malalignment or maltracking of the patella.

Machines can also be used to strengthen the knee, especially the leg extension (Fig. 15-11).

Lower Leg Injuries

Most lower leg injuries in recreational adults are overuse injuries of the muscle-tendon units. Careful evaluation must be done to determine the site of pain or tenderness. You should never be content with a diagnosis of shin splints. Activity-related pain in the athlete subject to repetitive micro-trauma activities, such as running, may indeed be a tendinitis, but it may also be a stress fracture of the tibia or even fibula, as well as compartment syndrome of one of the four muscle compartments of the lower leg.

The major muscles of the lower leg are contained in four different fascial envelopes which are relatively unyielding. They can form a constraining envelope about the muscles that can impair arterial inflow or venous out-flow if swelling occurs in the muscles contained in the compartment. These compartment syndromes are usually overuse injuries and are a result of inappropriate training techniques of the muscles involved. While they usu-ally are present as a slow, insidious, and activity-related pain in the involved compartment, they may also have an acute onset in association with activity and be a true emergency. If steps are not taken to relieve the pressure within the compartment or restore the blood flow and drainage of the compartment, death of muscle, tendon, and nerve elements contained within the compartment can occur, resulting in permanent impairment.

You can prevent most lower-extremity overuse injuries by slow, progressive training techniques. If an acute compartment syndrome devel-ops, however, you should be immobilized and your extremity elevated to the level of the heart, while ice is applied to the involved compartment. If symptoms do not rapidly abate and if pressure measurement of the involved compartment suggests significant elevation of compartment pressure, im-mediate surgical fascial release should be considered.

Several acute injuries to the lower-extremity musculature can occur in the recreational athlete. One of these, the tennis leg, is actually an acute tear of the medial head of the calf muscle from its subjacent tendon. Initiating symptoms can often be very debilitating. The diagnosis can usually be readily made by the localized site of the tenderness and swelling and often by the relative elevated level of the involved gastrocnemius muscle belly. Conservative management techniques are satisfactory for this injury, and full return to athletic activities can be anticipated.

The other acute injury that can occur in this area is a rupture of the tendo Achillis. This injury often occurs in racket sports. The injured athlete often describes a sensation similar to being hit in the back of the heel with a projectile. These ruptures are generally complete, with detachment of the proximal muscles and tendons from the os calcis (heel bone) below.

Table 15-2

	Injury To					
	Pelvis	**Hip**	**Thigh**	**Knee**	**Leg**	**Ankle-foot**
Archery	L	L	L	L	L	L
Automobile racing	M	M	M	M	M	M
Baseball	L	L	L	M	L	M
Basketball	L	L	L	M	L	M
Bicycling	L	L	L	L	L	L
Bowling	L	L	L	L	L	L
Diving	L	L	L	L	L	L
Football	H	H	H	H	H	H
Golf	L	L	L	L	L	L
Gymnastics	H	H	M	H	M	H
Handball	L	L	L	M	L	M
Hang gliding	H	H	H	H	H	H
Ice hockey	M	M	M	M	M	M
Ice-skating	M	M	M	M	L	M
Motorcycle racing	H	H	H	H	H	H
Racquetball	L	L	L	M	L	M
Roller-skating	M	M	M	M	L	M
Running	M	M	M	H	M	H
Skiing	M	M	M	M	M	M
Soccer	M	M	M	M	M	M
Squash	L	L	L	M	L	M
Swimming	L	L	L	M	L	L
Tennis	L	L	L	M	L	M
Water skiing	M	M	L	M	L	L
Weight lifting	M	M	M	M	L	M

L = low risk of injury   M = moderate risk of injury   H = high risk of injury

Figure 15–14

BONES OF THE FOOT

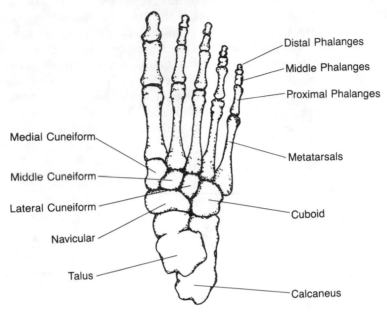

Distal Phalanges

Middle Phalanges

Proximal Phalanges

Medial Cuneiform

Middle Cuneiform

Lateral Cuneiform

Metatarsals

Navicular

Cuboid

Talus

Calcaneus

Exercises for the lower leg include stair climbing, walking on one's toes, toe lifts, jumping rope, and partial squats with weight on one's shoulders. All these exercises strengthen the gastrocnemius soleus musculature in the back of the leg. The tibialis anterior muscles in the front of the leg can be strengthened by extension of the foot with a sandbag or other weight on top of the foot.

Ankle and Foot

Your ankle and foot are designed primarily for strength, flexibility, and coordinated movement. Comprised of 26 bones (see Fig. 15-14), this structure is primarily responsible for absorbing the shock of weight bearing. The movements at the ankle include:

1. dorsi (upward) flexion—tibialis anterior, extensor digitorum longus, extensor hallucis longus, and peroneus tertius muscles (see Fig. 15-15).

2. plantar flexion—gastrocnemius, soleus, plantaris, peroneus longus and brevis, and tibialis posterior muscles.

Lateral motion of the foot mainly takes place at the subtalar joint. Your toes can move in flexion, extension, adduction, and abduction.

Injuries to the foot and ankle are common in recreational athletes. They

Figure 15–15

FOOT, MEDIAL ASPECT

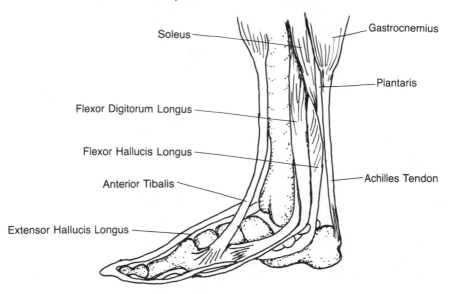

Soleus — Gastrocnemius

Plantaris

Flexor Digitorum Longus

Flexor Hallucis Longus

Anterior Tibialis — Achilles Tendon

Extensor Hallucis Longus

may be due to poor foot hygiene, improper footwear, or congenital faulty alignments. While many injuries are the result of recurrent microtrauma, most sprains are the result of single impact macrotrauma.

Ankle sprains are generally of the lateral collateral ligaments of the ankle. Localized swelling immediately subjacent to the medial malleolus and over the anterior aspect of the ankle joint, as well as swelling and ecchymosis (discoloration) below the site of injury, are common. Physical examination will generally confirm the diagnosis.

Debate exists as to the proper management of severe ligamentous derangements at the ankle. Most sports medicine physicians feel that acute repair of ligamentous disruption at the ankle is rarely indicated. Even in severe disruptions of a lateral ankle, as demonstrated by stress radiographs, many physicians will initiate treatment with a period of 7 to 10 days of cast immobilization, followed by early ambulation in a cast brace or special splint that allows flexion and extension of the ankle while limiting inversion and eversion.

As with any acute injury of soft tissues, rest, ice, compression, and elevation are indicated. It is particularly important in ankle injuries, however, to institute weight-bearing as early as possible in order to prevent progressive debilitation of the entire lower extremity. If heel-toe ambulation is not possible with soft dressings and crutch support, a short leg walking cast or cast brace should be used until it is possible. Subsequent

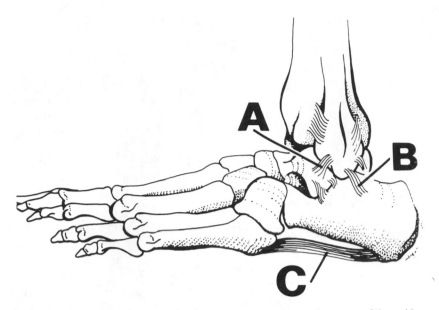

Figure 15–16. The foot and ankle. Sprain of the lateral collateral ligaments of the ankle are common. Less severe sprains involve the (**A**) fibulotalar ligaments, while more severe sprains involve both this ligament and the (**B**) fibulocalcaneal ligament. (**C**) Chronic plantar fascitis can be one of the most difficult injuries to treat, particularly in runners. Reproduced with permission from *Sports Medicine in Primary Care* by Robert C. Cantu, M.D. © 1982 D.C. Heath and Company.

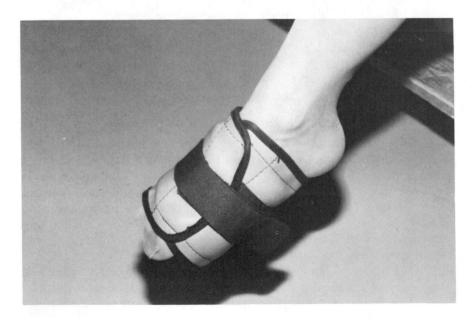

Figure 15–17. A foot exercise.

restoration of the strength and excursion of all the muscle-tendon units about the ankle, and in particular at the tendo Achillis, is important. Persistent tightness of the tendo Achillis after ankle sprain has been shown to be an important factor in reinjury.

In overuse injuries of the foot and ankle, careful attention to localization and diagnostic accuracy is essential. In the foot itself, tendinitis and stress fractures can be easily confused (Fig. 15-16). Stress fractures of the foot bones (metatarsals), especially the second metatarsals, are common overuse injuries, particularly in the runner.

An injury of particular concern in the runner, and one which can often present dramatic difficulty in management, is inflammation of the plantar fascia of the foot. The plantar fascia is a heavy fibrous structure extending from the base of the heel up to the mid-foot. It appears to be a functional component of the foot and ankle spring mechanism, and relative tightness of the plantar fascia is often associated with relative tightness of the heel cord and other structures at the back of the foot. Plantar fascitis is a tearing of this heavy fibrous structure, and the subsequent healing and scarring increase its tightness. The end result can be a pain syndrome localized on the bottom and outer aspect of the heel area, which can be very debilitating. Improvement can often be attained by the use of orthotics and even taping techniques, which prevent inward movement of the foot. Ultimate management often includes a satisfactory stretching and strength-

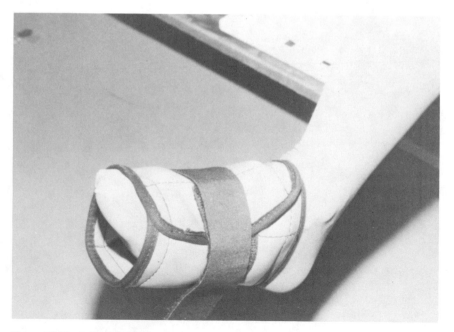

Figure 15–18. A foot exercise.

ening program for the small muscles of the foot as well as the plantar fascia. Where conservative techniques have failed, a surgical release of the plantar fascia and detachment of its fibers from the bony os calcis can give relief and allow resumption of its activities.

Exercises for the Foot and Ankle

The lower leg, foot, and ankle work largely as a unit. The same exercises can be used to strengthen all three areas. Some of the best include stair climbing, toe lifts, and partial squats with weights. Ankle flexion and extension can also be carried out with progressive increments of weight (Figs. 15-17 and 15-18). The same recommendations as for exercises elsewhere apply.

Chapter 16

Your Personal Sport-Specific Conditioning Program

In Chapter 4, you were given the information to design your own aerobic exercise prescription. Your aerobic exercise program includes a warm-up, a stimulus period, and a cool-down phase and depends on your present level of fitness and weight. In this chapter, we will discuss a supplementary weight-training and resistive exercise program that is sport-specific. We in sports medicine now realize that properly executed weight training not only enhances performance and rehabilitates from injury, but it also, and perhaps most important, protects against injury. This is also true for women and adolescents. While women and prepubertal youth will not demonstrate significant increase in muscle bulk due to the lack of testosterone, marked increases in strength are still seen with weight training.

At this point, I wish to make an unequivocal distinction between weight lifting, a sport I do not recommend for youth, women, or recreational adults, and weight training, which involves a series of progressive resistance exercises designed to attain speed, strength, and endurance. Weight lifting involves training to make one maximal lift and accordingly has a high risk of musculoskeletal injury. Weight training involves many repetitions (12 to 15) of progressively increasing weights that augment your speed, "explosive power," strength, and endurance.

Certain fundamentals should be followed in any weight-training program. First, you must understand the three types of contractions: isotonic, isometric, and isokinetic. Free weights are an example of isotonic exercises—the same weight through a range of motion. The machines are an example of isokinetic, or the same weight moved at a constant rate of speed through a full range of motion. Isometric, no movement, contractions are not recommended in the recreational adult, as the blood pressure is elevated by the Valsalva maneuver (carried out when you blow forcefully outwards against a resistance so that you can't let any air out), increasing the risk of heart attack or stroke. We now feel it is best to exercise muscles through their full range of motion for maximum benefit. Controversy persists as to whether free weights (isotonic) or the Nautilus and Universal machines (isokinetic) are best. The machines are safer and do not require a spotter. Ideally, if the isotonic free-weight lifts start from a position of on stretch and proceed at a constant rate of speed, about 1/5 maximum, they are equal to machines. In practice, this is usually difficult to do, as you tire toward the end of a set of repetitions and you tend to jerk the last few through. It is for this reason that I believe machines are safer. Machines are also a lot quicker to use than free weights, but this time may be more than offset by the fact that most people have to drive to a facility to use them. If they are available at work or where you normally play your sport, I recommend them over free weights as being safer and quicker. A general warm-up with stretching and full range of motion calisthenics should precede the weight-training exercises. A cooling-off period is also recommended.

Another important principle is to understand the concept of selecting a weight with which you complete 3 sets of 12 to 15 repetitions each, with a minute or two rest in between sets. When you can complete the third set with moderate ease, it is time to add another 5 pounds for the arms and 10 pounds for the legs and trunk.

Ideally, you should exercise a set of muscles, say your biceps and triceps, three times a week. If you prefer to work out every day, concentrate on different areas of the body (e.g., upper body, trunk, lower extremities) on different days of the week. The maximum number of sets should not be done while playing your sport and should be reserved for the "off season." This is because your muscle fibers are broken down by heavy lifting and it will hinder performance in your sport on that day. The three sets of repetitions are safe to pursue during the season, but it is not recommended on the day of a "big game" or match. In skill positions, like throwing for a football quarterback or baseball pitcher, it may be wise not to exercise the arms and shoulders during the season.

Proper breathing is important, as it assists in restabilizing the trunk musculature. You should inhale deeply just prior to starting a lift and exhale forcefully at the end of the lift as the return movement commences. This actually aids in carrying out the lift.

With these principles in mind, I have prepared in Table 16-1 a weight training program for each of our popular sports with a warm-up and cooling-off period included. Table 16-2 depicts some of the exercises to strengthen a particular area of the body. It is not suggested that every one need be done at each workout session. If you plan to exercise both the upper and lower body, select 12 to 14 exercises, say six for the lower body and eight for the upper body. In addition to this program, you can also receive benefit from carrying out the specific activity of your sport with a weighted object, as long as you can mimic the precise activity. Examples include strengthening a throwing arm by throwing a weighted ball, swinging

Table 16-1

	Warm-up	Neck	Shoulder	Upper arm, and elbow	Forearm, wrist, hand	Thorax	Abdomen	Hip	Knee	Lower leg, foot, ankle	Cool-down
	Any 5 exercises from pages 76–77	\<-- Isokinetic strength training -->									Any 5 exercises from pages 76–77
Archery			X	X	X						
Baseball			X	X	X	X	X	X	X	X	
Basketball			X	X	X	X	X	X	X	X	
Bowling			X	X	X	X					
Cycling							X	X	X	X	
Diving			X	X	X	X	X	X	X	X	
Football		X	X	X	X	X	X	X	X	X	
Golf							X	X			
Gymnastics		X	X	X	X	X	X	X	X	X	
Handball			X	X	X	X					
Hang gliding			X	X	X				X	X	X	
Ice hockey		X	X	X	X		X	X	X	X	
Ice-skating								X	X	X	
Lacrosse		X	X	X	X		X	X	X	X	
Motorcycle racing		X	X	X	X		X	X	X	X	
Racquetball			X	X	X		X	X	X	X	
Roller-skating								X	X	X	
Rowing			X	X	X		X	X	X	X	
Rugby		X	X	X	X		X	X	X	X	
Running			X	X		X	X	X	X	X	
Skiing			X		X		X	X	X	X	
Soccer		X	X					X	X	X	
Squash			X	X	X	X	X	X	X	X	
Swimming			X	X	X	X	X	X	X	X	
Tennis			X	X	X		X	X	X	X	
Volleyball			X	X	X		X	X	X	X	
Water skiing			X	X	X	X	X	X	X	X	
Weight lifting			X	X	X	X	X	X	X	X	
Wrestling		X	X	X	X	X	X	X	X	X	

a weighted bat or tennis racquet, or moving your arms in a particular
swimming stroke with a light dumbbell in each hand.

Archery

Archery is a skill sport that uses primarily your arms and shoulders for
strength and eyes to site your bow. To the extent you can easily pull a bow
at a higher poundage, performance may be enhanced. The major exercises
selected are, thus, those involving your arms and shoulders.

Baseball

Baseball demands a great deal of all-around ability including hand-eye
coordination, quickness of both hands and feet, power, and endurance.
The basic skills of hitting involve your hip, wrist, triceps, and shoulder
muscles. Running utilizes primarily your buttock and leg muscles, while
throwing uses your leg, hip, back, wrist, elbow, and shoulder muscles. In
the throwing motion, your shoulder and elbow are especially prone to
injury, and strength training will lessen the risk of injury.

Table 16-2

Area of Body	Exercise	Muscles Involved
Neck	shoulder shrug Fig. 14-5	trapezius, back of neck
	4-way machine	front, back, sides of neck
	Figs. 12-3 to 12-6	front, back, sides of neck
	turn against own	
	resistance Figs. 12-7 to	
	12-9	
Shoulder	push-up	pectorals, deltoids, triceps, biceps
	shoulder shrug Fig. 14-5	trapezius
	lateral raise and overhead	deltoids, triceps
	press	
	Figs. 14-6, 14-7a, b	
	overhead pull-down	latissimus dorsi, biceps
	Fig. 14-8	
	shoulder abductor	deltoids, trapezius
	Fig. 14-9	
	decline press Fig. 14-10	chest, shoulders, triceps
Upper arm and elbow	elbow flexion Fig. 14-18	biceps
	elbow extension	triceps
	Fig. 14-19	

Table 16-2 (continued)

Area of Body	Exercise	Muscles Involved
Upper arm and elbow	elbow supination Fig. 14-20	supinators, forearm
	elbow pronation Fig. 14-21	pronators, forearm
Forearm, wrist, hand	wrist curl Figs. 14-24, 25	
	wrist flexion Fig. 14-26	wrist flexors
	wrist extension Fig. 14-27	wrist extensors
	wrist supination Fig. 14-20	wrist supinators
	wrist pronation Fig. 14-21	wrist pronators
	hand squeeze Fig. 14-28	intrinsic hand muscles
Thorax	push-up	pectoralis major, triceps, deltoids
	bench press	pectoralis major, triceps, deltoids
	super pull-over	latissimus dorsi of back plus torso muscles
	double chest	pectoralis major, deltoid
Abdomen	sit-ups Fig. 13-1	rectus abdominus
	abdominal machine Fig. 13-2	rectus abdominus
Hip	flexion	iliopsoas
	extension Fig. 15-9	quadriceps, hamstrings
	abduction Fig. 15-8	abductors
	adduction Fig. 15-7	adductors
Knee	flexion Fig. 15-10	hamstrings
	extension Fig. 15-11	quadriceps
Lower leg, foot, ankle	stair climbing with weight	gastrocnemius
	toe lifts	gastrocnemius
	partial squats	gastrocnemius, quadriceps
	ankle extension Fig. 15-18	tibialis anterior
	ankle flexion Fig. 15-17	gastrocnemius

Numerous studies have shown that throwing speed, batting, and running speed can be improved by weight training. In addition to the exercises given, workouts swinging a weighted bat and throwing a weighted ball are recommended. A weighted baseball can be made by opening the seam of the baseball, drilling a ⅜- to ½-inch hole to the center of the ball, and filling this hole with several ounces of soft lead obtained at a plumbing or hardware supply store. The remainder of the hole is then filled with cotton and the cover resewn. A weighted bat can be prepared by drilling a 2-inch hole vertically in the end of the bat and filling it with about 5 ounces of lead. While it is emphasized that the weight-training program should be vigorously pursued only during the off season, the use of a weighted bat or ball can safely be pursued during the season. It is also my recommendation for a skill position like pitching that, during the season, resistance exercises for the torso, back, abdomen, and legs be used; the arm and shoulder are best exercised by the act of throwing, and their weight training is best left to the off season.

Basketball

Basketball has become increasingly more physical with considerable body contact. Quickness, jumping ability, and aggressiveness is especially sought. With the exception of the weighted bat and baseball, the same weight-training regimen for baseball players is appropriate for basketball players. The three primary skills are jumping (buttocks, quadriceps, hamstrings), throwing (latissimus dorsi, deltoids, triceps, pectorals), and dribbling (hand and wrist flexors). In addition to the weight-training exercises, passing and one- and two-handed shooting drills to a fellow athlete serves to strengthen the wrists, fingers, forearms, and shoulders. To further heighten explosive jumping, players will benefit from wearing a 5- to 10-pound weighted belt while practicing rebounds.

Cycling

Of all the areas in outdoor sports, none has enjoyed a greater surge than bicycling. Bicycling as a sport, a family recreation, and a serious means of transportation is becoming almost as popular in the United States as it is in Europe.

A vigorous, endurance-oriented sport, bicycling is a perfect combination of fitness activity and challenging sport. Bicycling's popularity has caused interest in training techniques for competitive as well as weekend bicyclists.

There are three means of improving ability. Compromising any of them will produce an athlete falling short of full potential. The athlete should (1) practice the skills needed, (2) learn effective strategies, and (3) improve physical efficiency. This last part is primarily in the improvement of cardiovascular fitness and the level of strength.

In the bicycling world, many cyclists do little or nothing to improve their strength. While they will build a certain amount of strength from riding a bike, it will not be enough to reach maximum potential. Cyclists sometimes fear an increase in strength will reduce their speed of movement, range of movement, or flexibility or in some other way limit their functional ability. These fears are without foundation.

Bowling

Bowling uses primarily your shoulder, arm, wrist, and hand muscles. Weight training will not only protect against injury and improve the velocity of your ball, but it will also guard against fatigue in tournament settings. For the serious bowler, this becomes very important and may be the margin between a successful and unsuccessful tournament season. For the once- or twice-a-week recreational bowler, a more aerobically oriented supplemental program would be more desirable.

Diving

Diving places the same physical demands on the body as does gymnastics. It combines explosive power with excessive flexibility. Maximal strength of the feet, ankles, and legs is essential, but so, too, is arm and trunk strength. Considerable extra attention to stretching drills to increase flexibility is also important.

Football

As one of the nation's most popular participant and spectator sports, football is played and watched by millions of people across the country every weekend during the season. The action on the gridiron is affected by a number of factors: the strategy employed by the opposing coaches, the inherent abilities of the two teams, and the collective dedication to *winning* exhibited by the individual players. One thing that affects all three of the aforementioned factors is the physical fitness level of the team members. A coach whose team is faster and stronger than his opponent's will develop a strategy to take advantage of his team's assets. A player who possesses a high level of personal fitness is better equipped to perform on the football field.

Individuals who are physically fit can translate their emotional commitment to winning into tangible performances on the gridiron. Without question, the primary fitness component for the football player is muscular fitness.

Muscular strength is the basis for every powerful, explosive movement made by a football player during a game. Muscular fitness also helps protect an athlete against the possibility of injuries. Not only do stronger muscles enable the football player to block and tackle better, run faster, and kick and run farther, but they also provide increased joint stability, thus protecting the vulnerable neck, shoulder, elbow, wrist, hip, knee, and ankle joints. In addition, muscular strength improves the performance of a football player by increasing the endurance level of the many muscles utilized during a game. A high degree of muscular endurance enables a football player to minimize the muscular fatigue that so frequently limits athletic performance.

To some degree, a majority of all football players and coaches recognize the role that muscular strength plays in developing a successful team. As a result, most teams engage in strength-training programs of some sort. A large number of these programs, however, do not achieve the best results possible, especially considering the time and effort put into these programs by everyone involved. Faulty training techniques and a lack of under-standing of the basic principles of exercise are the typical reasons for such a shortcoming.

Although virtually all of an individual's muscles are used when playing football, weight training programs for the football players should concentrate on developing strong shoulders, arms, the lower back, and upper legs. Likewise, the muscular development program for a football player should strengthen the neck, increase joint stability, and increase and maintain the joint flexibility required to prevent serious injuries. In addition to weight training, punters and kickers can benefit from practicing the high-kick while wearing weighted shoes. A weighted football weighing 3 to 4 pounds can also be made from unlacing a football, removing the air bladder, and stuffing it with cotton or sponge rubber. Passing and centering the weighted ball will strengthen the arm, wrist, finger, and shoulder muscles used by quarterbacks and centers.

Golf

Power in golf comes primarily from your upper extremities, especially your forearms, wrists, and hands. Golf also involves a great deal of "touch." There is no question that you can add power to your drives by utilizing weight training, especially to your forearms and wrists. During the golf season, however, such training should be modest so that fluidity of swing and touch are not sacrificed.

The follow-through in golf, especially with the driver, places stresses on the back due to the hyperextended twisted position assumed at the end of your swing. Thus, to protect against back injury, I suggest you carry out one or more of the abdominal exercises all year.

Gymnastics

Every portion of the body is exercised during gymnastic routines. Your strength-training exercises, like your warm-up and cool-down exercises, should thus involve all major muscle groups of the body. In addition, sit-ups wearing a weighted belt around the abdomen or on an incline board are recommended. Vaulters may also benefit from wearing a weighted belt, and all gymnasts will benefit from chinning with such a belt.

Handball

The upper extremities are maximally stressed during handball, and thus your performance and safety will be enhanced by a strength-training regimen to that area of the body. Handball requires a great deal of aerobic fitness, and while I have nothing against resistance training for your lower body, your time might best be spent running. Handball also places stresses on your lower back because of the quick movements required, as you often reach backward placing your low back in extension. Thus, I have included the abdominal exercises as well. The conditioning program for handball is similar for the racket sports, such as racquetball, paddle tennis, squash, and tennis.

Hang Gliding

Hang gliding and sky diving are two of the most hazardous recreational pursuits. Deaths occur even among the most experienced practitioners. The "sport" of hang gliding utilizes primarily your upper body while flying and your lower body while landing. Each area will, therefore, profit from strength training, primarily in a protective manner for your legs.

Ice-Skating

Ice-skating requires the same lower extremity and cardiovascular demands as ice hockey. Since there is no stick-handling or body contact, singles skating does not require upper body conditioning. If one is involved in pairs skating, however, total body strength training, exclusive of the neck, is recommended.

Lacrosse

Proficiency in the sport of lacrosse requires a high level of *total* fitness and a mastery of a wide variety of skills. It is a physically demanding sport with a great deal of running and ruggedness to withstand, with little protective equipment, and forceful body contact.

Lacrosse requires that the athlete possess stamina, muscular fitness, flexibility, and an extensive array of motor abilities. Adequate stamina enables the individual to meet the cardiovascular demands imposed by this fast-moving sport. Muscular fitness has an effect on almost every aspect of lacrosse: shooting, stick control, body checking, running, and (perhaps most important) preventing muscular fatigue. Since flexibility and joint stability play an important role in the success of a lacrosse player, improvement in these factors should be given adequate attention in every lacrosse player's conditioning program. This attention not only will affect the lacrosse player's performance on the field, but will also decrease the possibility of incurring an injury. A lacrosse player should combine a total body weight-training program and a vigorous running program with optimum flexibility training in the warm-up and cooling-off periods.

211

Motorcycle Racing

Primarily because forceful contact with the ground, haybale, or both is inevitable for those who race motorcycles, total body conditioning is advisable to minimize the risk of injury. Such conditioning will also improve endurance, something especially important to motorcross, a physically demanding variant of motorcycle racing.

Racquetball

Racquetball is a fast-moving, high intensity, physically demanding activity. Speed of movement, explosive power, hand-eye coordination, and the ability to maintain these attributes at a high level during the course of a match are essential skills of the successful racquetballer. Conditioning for racquetball, therefore, encompasses sharpening the following factors: endurance, strength, speed, agility, flexibility, and coordination. While playing the game itself is probably the best "overall" conditioner for the racquetballer, a properly planned conditioning program should augment the time spent on the court playing.

Running should be included in any conditioning program for racquetball. Depending on the athlete's devotion to the game, the conditioning regimen will vary from a few long-distance runs of 2 to 3 miles to a demanding program combining distance runs, interval work, and sprint workouts. The long runs are included to develop the aerobic capacity required to play those extended three-game matches, while the sprint training helps develop the quickness needed for explosive movements on the court. The interval work benefits both speed and endurance. Skipping rope should also be included in the running program in order to improve quickness and agility

All conditioning routines should include some form of stretching or flexibility exercises. Racquetball is no exception. Increased flexibility will not only improve the athlete's on-the-court performance, but will also improve his chances of avoiding injuries. Before and after both workouts and games are the best times to stretch or loosen up. Of particular concern to the racquetballer are the muscles of the legs, lower back, and racquet arm. Flexibility exercises need be no more elaborate than toe or straddle stretches and leg pullovers from the supine position, but they should be of the static stretch variety in which the muscles and joints are loosened by the individual's body weight, not by bouncing movements.

Muscular development is essential both to a racquetballer's overall performance on a court and to help prevent injuries. The player deficient in muscular fitness will normally observe a gradual reduction in his performance level during the course of a prolonged match or tournament. Development of strength in the muscles used to run and to hit the ball helps to prevent or minimize injury to such areas as the knees, shoulders, and elbow of the dominant arm. In addition, greater strength increases the athlete's ability to move quickly and to hit with power.

212

Roller-Skating

Roller-skating places considerable physical stresses on your lower extremities and does require a degree of aerobic fitness as well. The same statements apply for this sport as for ice-skating, as regards both singles and doubles competition.

Rowing

This is one of our most physically demanding sports, requiring extreme cardiovascular and musculoskeletal fitness. A running program will aid in developing the cardiovascular system while training will enhance musculoskeletal fitness. In addition, interval training techniques, rowing at tempos and time intervals faster than normally used in competition, will enhance performance. You can use arm and ankle weights in your rowing conditioning program as well.

Rugby

The physical demands made on rugby players are quite similar to football. It is slightly more of an aerobic sport, but a strength-training program for rugby would be the same as for footall.

Running

Running has become an increasingly popular form of exercise. Its appeal is not limited by age, sex, occupation, or any other factor. It can be a great, inexpensive way to improve your health.

Running holds a variety of levels, from the neighborhood jogger to the serious marathon competitor. As more and more runners have become involved, it has become clear that uninformed runners can harm their bodies if they are not careful. It is not prudent to put on some footwear and start running. Tremendous advances in footwear design have been made in the past few years. Therefore, a runner should take advantage of this knowledge and select proper footwear.

Resistance training is also important for runners, since it improves strength and increases resistance to injury, leading to improved performance. Resistance training produces stronger muscles, which stabilize joints and protect crucial ligaments. The runner's weight-bearing joints are better protected as well. Women runners have a potential for the development of pelvic injuries due to the skeletal make-up and the stress running puts on it. Resistance training can lessen the potential by strengthening the musculature.

Performance improvement as a result of resistance training is closely linked to strength and freedom from injuries. Prolonged good breathing will delay the onset of fatigue. When the upper body is in a more upright position, the chest cavity rises and falls more efficiently, allowing more effective breathing. Your intercostal muscles between the ribs, the diaphragm, and erectors along the spine may be strengthened with torso and abdominal resistance exercises. Upper body strength also provides for a more effective elbow drive.

Interval training should be employed as part of any running conditioning program, as tip-top aerobic conditioning requires giving your cardiovascular system workloads beyond previously established threshholds. This results in greater endurance. This essentially involves the same overload principle to your cardiovascular system that weight training employs with your muscles.

There are four components in interval training: (1) a particular distance that is run at a (2) predetermined space and (3) repeated a prescribed number of times with a (4) precise recovery period during which you jog leisurely between repetitions. Interval training should not be done more than once every three days and ideally should commence many months before the competitive season commences. Most feel the pace, recovery, period, and distance should be kept constant with the number of repetitions increased as endurance increases. Others will argue, however, that both distance and repetitions can be increased to best increase endurance.

An adjunct but not an alternative to interval training involves "fortlek" or literally "speed play." Originating in Sweden, this type of cross-country training involves running at varying paces over varying terrain. Designed to avoid boredom while enhancing stamina and strength, this is an excellent off-season conditioner or adjunct to interval training. Because it does not allow you to acquire pace judgment as well as interval training, it is not suggested to the exclusion of interval training.

Skiing

This is both a mentally and physically demanding sport. Skiing places heavy stresses especially on your hips and knees. The muscles that are most important to skiing are those in the legs that produce the side-to-side and rotating movements required to initiate turns. When these muscles do not have an adequate level of development (particularly at the beginning of the season), the skier is frequently forced to utilize a pivital movement of the hips or the upper body to start the skis turning. This adjustment not only makes for a delayed turn, it also keeps the individual's skiing pleasure to a minimum because he or she does not have total, confident control of the skis. Consequently, it is obvious that the time spent in the exercise room will reward the skier many times over by allowing the individual to start his ski season prepared for challenges of the slope. Alpine skiing also requires a great deal of flexibility; hence, in addition to strength training, a broad program of stretching and general flexibility exercises are recommended. Cross-country skiing requires greater upper body strength and aerobic fitness. Cardiorespiratory fitness must be stressed, either with an off-season program of running or roller skiing. The knee is the most vulnerable joint the poor category received low scores for endurance, calorie consumption, and strength.

Those sports that are in the fair group generally had several factors where they scored a 1 and, thus, removed themselves from the good group. Diving scored poorly on endurance, calorie consumption, and hand-eye coordination. Football scored poorly on cost and injury risk. Ice-skating and roller-skating received low ratings on cost, hand-eye coordination, and convenience. Rowing scored poorly on agility, convenience, and hand-eye coordination. Cost, convenience, and injury risk prevented Alpine skiing from attaining a higher ranking. Actually, the cost for Alpine skiing and automobile racing so far exceeded any other pursuit, that I toyed with the idea of giving them a zero under that criterion instead of the minimal 1.

Those sports that attained a good rating generally attained mostly 2 and occasional 3 scores for all 10 criteria. The reason racquetball and squash did not join handball in the excellent group is their greater risk of injury, not only from the ball that travels faster off a racket, but especially from the racket itself. Swimming, undoubtedly one of the best aerobic pursuits and total body conditioners, failed to rank higher because of the low scores for agility and hand-eye coordination. If you have convenient access to a pool year round and enjoy swimming, though, I would have no aversion to your pursuing swimming as your exercise pursuit. With the water supporting your body weight and eliminating jarring pressures on your musculoskeletal system, swimming has one of the lowest risks of injury of any sport.

Generally, those sports that received an excellent rating were good to excellent on all criteria with no glaring weaknesses. Soccer is the one exception, and may have led the list, were it not for its low score in hand-eye coordination. Basketball, described by Tom Heinsohn, a former player and coach of the Boston Celtics, as "a game that is a combination of ballet and wrestling," and lacrosse, now the most popular school spring sport in the mid-Atlantic and northeast regions, were the only team sports to make the excellent category. Cross-country skiing would have scored even higher were it not for the convenience factor and the fact that you cannot pursue it year round in most regions. If you were to couple cross-country skiing with roller skiing, its snowless equivalent, this combination would lead the list.

The Ideal Combination

Your exercise program, of course, can consist of different sports on different days of the week. By pursuing such a mixed program, your risk of overuse injuries is minimized. One of the very best combinations is running 3 or 4 days a week combined with a Nautilus or other resistive exercise program 3 days a week. For those who have orthopedic conditions that makes running difficult or for those who do not enjoy running, a cycling-resistive exercise program makes an essentially equally effective combination. If such a combination is pursued, the two pursuits should ideally be followed on alternate days with stretching every day. Thus, resistive exercises on Monday, Wednesday, Friday, and running on Tuesday, Thursday, and Saturday, with Sunday off, would be an ideal combination.

Obviously work, travel, family obligations, and a host of other unforeseen emergencies will prohibit such a schedule from being religiously adhered to. Nonetheless, moderate compliance coupled with a positive lifestyle as discussed in Chapter 2 will afford you maximal health, energy, vitality, and positive self-image.

Sigmund Freud talked about work and love as being at the heart of health. I believe optimum health comprises a triangle that includes not only work and love, but exercise that is fun so that it becomes play. May you play lifelong!

Peace

Other Books by Dr. Robert C. Cantu

1. Cantu, R.C., *Toward Fitness.* Human Sciences Press, New York, N.Y., 1980.

2. Cantu, R.C., *Health Maintenance Through Physical Conditioning.* Wright-PSG Publishing Inc., Littleton, Mass., 1981.

3. Cantu, R.C., *The Exercising Adult.* The Collamore Press, D.C. Heath Company, Lexington, Mass., 1981.

4. Cantu, R.C., *Sports Medicine In Primary Care,* The Collamore Press, D.C. Heath Company, Lexington, Mass., 1982.

5. Cantu, R.C., *Diabetes Prevention and Control Through Exercise.* E.P. Dutton, New York, N.Y., 1982.

6. Cantu, R.C., *Sports Medicine—Sports Science: Bridging the Gap.* The Collamore Press, D.C. Heath Co., Lexington, Mass., 1982.

7. Cantu, R.C., *Regaining Health and Fitness.* The Stephen Greene Press, Brattleboro, Vermont, 1982.